P9-BZO-392

Eat, Drink, and Be GORGEOUS

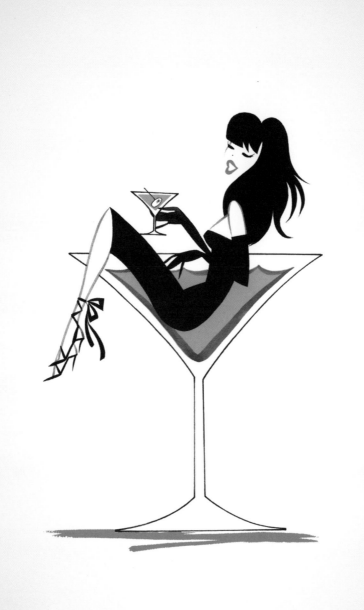

Eat, Drink, and Be GORGEOUS

A Nutritionist's Guide to Living Well While Living It Up

BY ESTHER BLUM, MS, RD, CDN, CNS

ILLUSTRATIONS BY JAMES DIGNAN

CHRONICLE BOOKS
SAN FRANCISCO

Text copyright © 2007 by Esther Blum.
Illustrations copyright © 2007 by James Dignan.
All rights reserved. No part of this book may be reproduced
in any form without written permission from the publisher.

Library of Congress Cataloging-in-Publication Data available.

ISBN: 978-0-8118-5540-2

Manufactured in China

Designed by Jillian Moffett Design, San Francisco

10 9 8 7

Chronicle Books LLC
680 Second Street
San Francisco, California 94107

www.chroniclebooks.com

No book can replace the services of a trained physician, and you should always consult with
your doctor for questions relating to your health. Every effort has been made to present the
information in this book in a clear, complete, and accurate manner; however, not every situation
can be anticipated, and the information in this book cannot take the place of a medical analysis
of your particular health and needs. Do not use any information contained in this book to make
a diagnosis, treat a health problem, or replace a doctor's judgment. Following tips or recommendations does not ensure that you will be healthy. Your health is the result of many factors,
some of which are not yet fully understood. It is important that you rely on only the personal
advice of a health-care professional to advise you on your specific situation. The author and
Chronicle Books hereby disclaim any and all liability resulting from injuries or damage caused
by following any recommendations contained in this book.

Advil is a registered trademark of Wyeth. Amstel Light is a registered trademark of Amstel Brouwerij B.V. Ben & Jerry's is a registered
trademark of Ben & Jerry's Homemade, Inc. Bisquick is a registered trademark of General Mills, Inc. Bud Light, Budweiser, and
Michelob Ultra are registered trademarks of Anheuser-Busch, Inc. Cinnabon is a registered trademark of Cinnabon, Inc. Coke, Diet
Coke, Diet Sprite, Diet Vanilla Coke, and Sprite are registered trademarks of the Coca-Cola Co. Coors Light is a registered trademark
of Coors Global Properties, Inc. Dos Equis is a registered trademark of CCM IP, S.A. Duncan Hines is a registered trademark of
the Procter & Gamble Co. Guinness Extra Stout is a registered trademark of Guinness PLC. Heineken is a registered trademark of
Heineken Brouwerijen B.V. Hershey's is a registered trademark of Hershey Chocolate & Confectionery Corp. Jack Daniel's is a registered trademark of Jack Daniel's Properties, Inc. Kahlúa is a registered trademark of the Kahlúa Co. M&M's, Milky Way, and Snickers
are registered trademarks of Mars, Inc. Miller Light and Miller Genuine Draft are registered trademarks of the Miller Products Co. Neti
pot is a registered trademark of the Himalayan International Institute of Yoga Science and Philosophy of the USA. Newcastle Brown
Ale is a registered trademark of Scottish & Newcastle PLC. Red Bull is a registered trademark of Red Bull GmbH. Samuel Adams is
a registered trademark of BBC Brands, LLC. Schlitz Light is a registered trademark of Jos. Schlitz Brewing Co. Tylenol is a registered
trademark of the Tylenol Co. Vital Choice is a registered trademark of Vital Choice Seafood, Inc.

FOR JEREMY, MY COMPASS STAR.

CONTENTS

FOREWORD

You've heard people talk about "the feel-good book of the year"? Well, *Eat, Drink, and Be Gorgeous* is "the feel-gorgeous book of the year"! This book is a triple-espresso wake-up call to tell us ladies that taking care of our oh-so-womanly selves can be oh-so-glam, and empower us to take full, feisty control of our health and diet. I consider this book to be a portable trainer, nutritionist, life coach, best friend, and fairy godmother all squooshed into one.

As a New York City girl, I didn't think it was possible for me to live a healthy lifestyle without missing out on all of life's fun. So when I met Esther, I joyously gobbled up and relished every bite of her bountiful advice on how I could be my most *she*donistic self without harming my body. Now I can party without the post-party depression, and I can drink like a pro—without all those cons. It's great to be a naughty girl while being nice to my body, hormones, and skin.

I used to joke, "If I gorge on all the foods I love, will that make me gorgeous?" Today, I say, gorge on this book. On the following pages, Esther dishes vice advice; she outlines the fabulous treats that can boost your system when you need it most (such as after a cocktail bender or a broken heart); and, best of all, she offers up sweet little tips on what to eat to rev up your engine in the bedroom.

Esther gives you the inside story on your inside's story. You'll learn why things work the way they work—and how to make sure your body has the best work ethic! Esther will show any woman—from the highly suburban to the wily urban—how to feel and be gorgeous from the inside out, so your vital organs will be just as fit as your toosh. *Eat, Drink, and Be Gorgeous* is perfect reading over cocktails or wheatgrass juice.

I wish Esther had been there for me in my twenties, to guide me through all of the magazine articles, useless diets, gnawing insecurities, and personal questions I had back then. But I'm delighted to have her now. Not only is she a nutritionist guru, but she's also a muckraker of sorts, leading the way for women to make the most of life's pleasures—without the guilt, or the hangovers, or the cellulite. The revelations in her book are surprising, fascinating, and, best of all, wildly useful. By the time you've finished this bible for the gorgeous, you'll have all the inside information you need to live life to the maximum, while keeping your weight, cholesterol, and remorse to a minimum. I can't wait to give this book to every sassy gal I know.

Now, if you will excuse me, I need to go grab some flax seed and a martini and be on my way.

Karen Salmansohn
Best-selling author of *Hot Mama* and *How To Be Happy, Dammit*

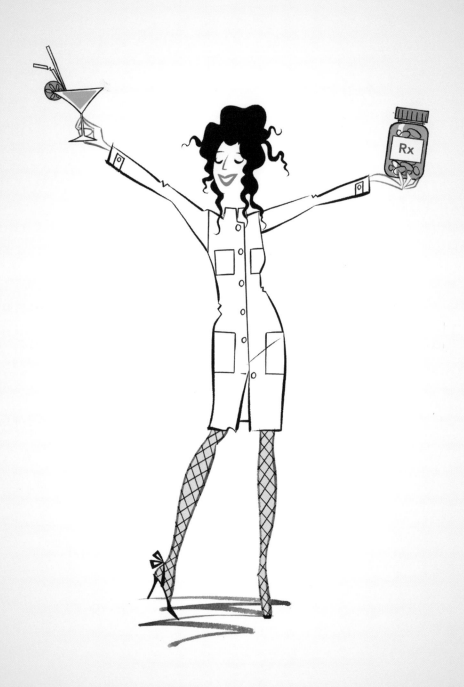

Introduction:
HELLO, GORGEOUS!

YOUR BODY MAY BE A TEMPLE, BUT WHO SAYS IT CAN'T BE A NIGHTCLUB?

In a perfect world, we gorgeous gals wear silk robes and marabou mules. We go to the swankest clubs, drink our martinis straight up, and meet fabulous people while looking absolutely radiant. The next morning we wake with the sun and head off to yoga class—with boundless energy and our skin aglow.

Sound like a dream come true? I'm here to tell you that all this can be yours. Well, I can't guarantee the silk robes and marabou slippers. But I can promise a gorgeous path to enlightenment. The sort of enlightenment I'm talking about means freedom from hangovers, guaranteed great sex, and the know-how to live it up without letting yourself go!

As your nutrition guru and food fashionista, I solemnly swear to teach you all my best-kept secrets. You'll learn how to be at your personal best whether you're out with the girls, out on a date, or (God forbid) down in the dumps post-breakup. I'll show you how to cook in the kitchen and cook in the bedroom. You'll find out how to balance gorgeous eating and drinking with a healthy lifestyle, and how to balance your hormones each month. Most important, I'm going to free you from the bonds of diet tyranny and teach you how to stop the chain reaction of pesky conditions that can put a damper on your health, your social life, and your sex life. You'll learn how to eat right and keep your body beautiful from the inside out. You'll learn how to fend off colds and flus, PMS, yeast infections, hangovers, and many other health-challenging conditions. You'll come away with your very own personal instruction book on how to keep your body running like a well-oiled machine so you can get on with your life and get out on the dance floor.

Get ready for the most delicious cocktail of wild fun, good health, and positive energy! *Eat, Drink, and Be Gorgeous* gives you all the ingredients. All you'll have to do is pour them into a shaker, add ice, a little spice ... *et voilà!* A naughty girl's drink to badness ... all while being soooo good.

STOP THE INSANITY!

At one time or another, we've all struggled with a negative body image and poor eating habits. It is not easy to juggle work, your social life, dating, and, most important, time for yourself. And the truth is, we even give each other some fierce competition in the land of self-confidence. The pressures we face today are greater than ever; they leave us little time to properly feed our emotional hungers, let alone our physical ones. We wear bras, corsets, panties, and shoes that painfully pinch us, suck us in, pull us up, and make us uncomfortable. So why would we want to read a book that does the same thing? That's not the reason you're reading this book, and it's definitely not why I wrote it!

This is not a diet book, and it does not contain any strict guidelines. I'm here to educate and empower you to make better choices for yourself while treating yourself with gentle loving-kindness—that's all! Read the book, chew on it, and when you're ready for a new challenge, you can incorporate as few or as many of these recommendations as you like. Every small change you incorporate into your lifestyle will make a big difference.

THE PATH TO ENLIGHTENMENT

In my fifteen years of nutritional counseling I have helped countless women adopt healthful lifestyles for themselves without losing out on all of the fun—cocktail parties, dinner dates, martinis, nightclubs, and sexcapades. I show my clients how to lead healthier lives *and* I encourage their naughty ways! I am pro-supplements, and I am pro-cosmopolitans. *Eat, Drink, and Be Gorgeous* compiles all of the secrets I have been sharing with my incredible clients for years. In fact, it is the book I wish someone had written for me when I was in my twenties. Back then I didn't have the knowledge or insight to make the connections between diet, supplements, physical and emotional health, and a healthy body image.

This book was inspired by my clients, colleagues, and friends, who encouraged me over the years to write down my sage words of wisdom. I wanted to do better and add some fun into the mix. We show off our best assets when we go out on the town in a sexy outfit; I'm bringing you a nutrition book with the same provocative packaging. Beauty and brains meet on these pages to make nutrition seductive, sensual, sophisticated, and sane. You get the best of both worlds here.

As a nutritionist and a resident of the city that never sleeps, I can personally attest to the benefits of the protocols I've laid out here. I've included something in this book for everyone, whether you are newly single and reinventing your lifestyle or are fully committed, on the go, and need to take a moment to recharge your batteries. I have taken my years of expertise and filtered out all the riffraff and the gunk so I can present you with a very pristine picture of what will get you through the good times and the bad. It's amazing what a difference good nutrition can make in your ability to handle stress while navigating through careers, dating, mating, and relating!

Your twenties and thirties are the best years to build the foundation for a house of good health. Picking up some good habits now will pay you back in kind years down the road. I attribute my good skin and healthy glow to a clean diet that I follow about 80 percent of the time; the other 20 percent I nourish my wild side. When I'm old and gray, I'd much rather have crinkles around my eyes from smiling than lines around my mouth from frowning, worrying about all my regrets in life! I don't want to be some old, farty grandma—I want to be a hip and sassy glam-ma! And I want the same for you, my darlings. That is why I'm here to teach you the best way to eat, drink, and be gorgeous.

It's time to get the party started. Powder on some body shimmer, slick on some gloss, freshen up your cocktail, and give your hair a tousle. Life awaits us—let's go!

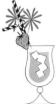

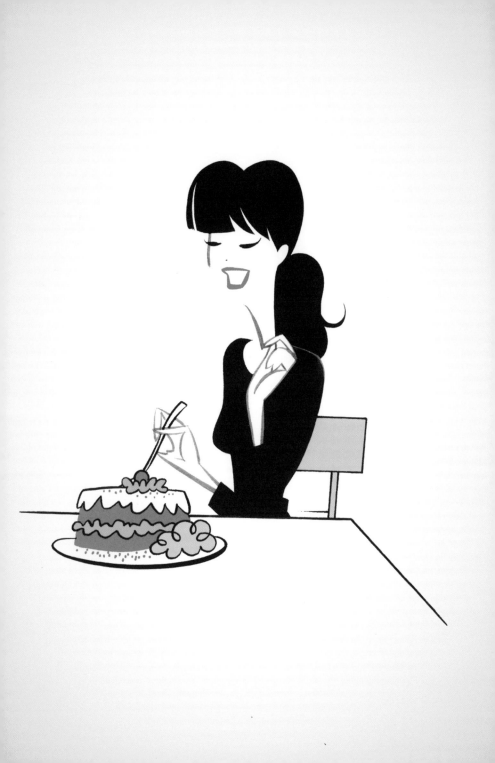

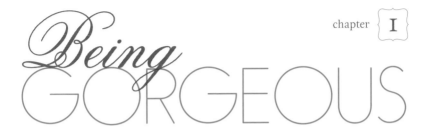

chapter I

Beauty is not caused. It is. – Emily Dickinson

Before we get started, I want to say one thing: This book is not about strict diets. *Non, non, ma petite coquette!* I'm not going to demand that you eliminate entire food groups or tell you that you can no longer eat past 5 P.M. Instead, *Eat, Drink, and Be Gorgeous* is all about moderation. It's about having your cake and eating it too (so to speak)!

But perhaps you're looking for a dominatrix who will spank you every time you've been naughty. Someone who will demand perfection, berating you into living a more submissive and Spartan lifestyle. Someone who will outline a program that will require you to cut out sinful foods and shed weight. If so, this book isn't for you. There is no way in hell I am going to put you through that torture or nonsense! *Au contraire, ma cherie*; I am going to do quite the opposite. I am going to empower you to be decadent and healthy at the same time. In this book, I'm going to give you little tools that you can pull out of your rhinestone-studded tool belt when desperate times call for desperate measures. And I'm going to teach you how to navigate life's land mines and prevent you from falling from grace when you're wearing three-inch stilettos.

Before we embark upon this journey, take a look at the list below. It outlines exactly what *Eat, Drink, and Be Gorgeous* will teach you. These lessons may seem somewhat unconventional—especially if you're one of those on-a-diet-all-the-time-and-always-deprived young babes. But as your nutritional fairy godmother, I promise you they will only enhance your life.

Eat, Drink, and Be Gorgeous will:

- Teach you how to have fun, go out, and be healthy—all at the same time
- Show you how to put the fun back in eating and avoid restricting yourself
- Get your groove back in the sack and get your mojo going
- Tell you the secrets of the nutritional it girls... and how they can help you
- Teach you what vitamins are right for you
- Empower you with the secrets of how to recover from a nasty hangover
- Help you realize that life is too short to be on a diet the whole time!

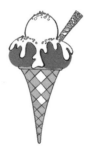

FILL-OSOPHY

If your mission is to add some health in your life, you must make it as enjoyable as possible. Would you rather work out at the gym or play out at the roller disco? Would you rather eat a bowl of diet Jell-O or a bowl of chocolate ice cream? If you approach your eating lifestyle with fun, passion, and creative energy, you will carry that same enthusiasm across all realms of your life. If you're passionate about eating and bring sensuality to it, you can imagine how well that will carry over into, ahem, *other* aspects of your life! And, ultimately, that is the goal I have for you. After all, if you're not having fun, what's the bloody point?

WE'VE COME A LONG WAY, BABY

The dietitian in today's society has it much better than the older generations did. When I first started out in the field, I had the impression that all
dietitians wore hairnets and stirred giant vats of soup, advocating the four
food groups and the merits of the food pyramid. Fortunately, the only nets we
wear today are fishnets; instead of stirring soup, we shake up martinis; and
the four food groups have fallen by the wayside, replaced by a more well-
rounded approach. Of course, in my house there are still four food groups:
chocolate, cocktails, desserts, and caffeine. (Kidding. Kidding!)

While dietitians have always advocated that diet is the absolute foundation of health, I'm here to tell you that pleasure is the most important nutrient in your diet. I've had many patients who are thin but absolutely miserable
because their eating fears and obsessions weigh on their psyches, pull them
down, and gnaw away at their esteem. On the other hand, I also have patients
who are five to ten pounds over their dream weight, yet live happy, fulfilling
lives because they aren't obsessing over every little morsel they put in their
mouths. Who's having more fun here despite a few extra pounds on her
frame?

Take a look at me. I don't have the perfect body, and like every other
woman out there, I have areas that I would like to improve upon. However,
I also enjoy eating gooey chocolate desserts and am famous for being the
vodka queen who makes some of the meanest martinis in town! If you told
me I could never enjoy these delights again, I would not enjoy my life to the
degree I do. Now, I don't indulge in these foods on a daily basis, but when I
have a craving, I give in to it. It helps balance my life and reminds me that I
need to have fun on a regular basis. This fun and free attitude carries over to
my nutrition practice as well. That is why I will never ask you to follow a plan
I couldn't follow myself.

Personally, I believe it's essential to eat a healthful diet, but if that's
not a reality for you right now, it's better to be honest with yourself. Make
slow and gradual changes rather than drastic, impermanent ones. Just like
weight loss, the slower you go, the more likely it is that you'll be successful
in sticking to it in the long run. Remember, my pretty perfectionistas: No
unforgiving diets are allowed in this book, nor will they be tolerated. There

is no place for self-flagellation, harsh criticisms, judgments, obsessions with thinness, or unworthiness here! Push those thoughts of doubt and fear out the window. Instead, focus on what makes you fabulous, babelicious, bootylicious, tatalicious, and toast yourself, darling! *You* are what makes you fabulous. Forget about those women's magazines that put skinny models on the cover. Remind yourself that the publishers of those mags prey on our insecurities. Being gorgeous is not about emulating an emaciated model. It's about learning about how to nourish your soul with fun and good health.

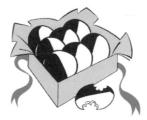

THE BLACK-AND-WHITE COOKIE: IS IT ALL OR NOTHING?

Life is a smorgasbord and most people are starving. —Mame

New York City is filled with all kinds of swingers. There are swingers who trade lovers, swing dancers on Broadway, and swinging singles. Then there are the diet swingers who come into my office every week. Those creatures I will affectionately call my little black-and-white cookies.

Now, if you're not familiar with a black-and-white cookie, you're in for a treat. I myself had never heard of a black-and-white cookie until my twenties, despite the fact that they are one of the last bastions of old New York deli culture. A sweet, chewy sugar cookie lies beneath the perfect yin-yang balance of chocolate and vanilla frostings. Just sinking your chompers into one can make you see God. And how a person eats the cookie can be a good window into how she eats in general.

So many of us are black-and-white about our eating habits. We will eat either the vanilla (angelic and wholesome) side or the chocolate (sinful and decadent) side, but not both. The same goes for our day-to-day diets: We're either "very good" all week or "very, very bad"! Our inner pendulum wildly swings back and forth. One week we're in the food equivalent of Las Vegas, indulging in over-the-top rich foods and drink; the next week we're at the monastery denying ourselves. You may even hear yourself say, "That will be the last cookie"—or doughnut or French fry or chip—"I ever eat. *Ever!*" Then you'll eat salads for one day. Maybe even two. By the third day, you'll never want to chew another vegetable again. It's straight for the cookie aisle you head, to devilishly devour those glorious treats. And then it's back to the drawing board all over again.

This all too familiar cycle is exhausting and self-defeating. I'm here to tell you that it doesn't have to be this way. The secret to keeping it all in balance is to eat right up the center of the cookie—that is, give yourself a little bit of what you crave. You see, I don't believe people can exist only in the land of black and white; I think we really need to play in the gray areas these days. I once had a patient who told me she constantly craved chocolate. So I said, "Well, how do you get rid of your cravings?" She said, "I eat chocolate!" My kind of girl. It's this sort of attitude that keeps us from the cycle of bingeing and denying.

In my experience, people eat the way they live and live the way they eat. So, my little vixen—have a sensual experience every time you pop a piece of food in your mouth. Savor the flavor, love each luscious bite, and be present in the moment.

If you take only one thing away from *Eat, Drink, and Be Gorgeous*, take this: It's okay to indulge in rich, delicious food—just as long as you indulge moderately. Now repeat the following mantras after me:

I will not restrict myself.

I will not deprive myself.

I will feed my physical and emotional hungers.

I will never starve myself again!

Simply put, that's what healthy eating is all about.

Here's a success story: I used to be very black-and-white in my outlook on life. I had perfectionist habits and was very hard on myself about getting things right. After living this way most of my life, I began to take a closer look at what a waste of time that was, and began to be true to myself. I quickly saw the rewards of living in the gray spaces and found that it set me free. Once I learned that I didn't have to be perfect, I started having a lot more fun! My new mantra became "It's not perfect, but it's perfect for me."

THE PLEASURE PRINCIPLE

What would happen if we gave ourselves permission to eat whatever we wanted but stopped eating when we were full? We'd be a hell of a lot more satisfied and would really enjoy our food. And by giving ourselves permission to eat whatever we wanted, we'd empower ourselves to have control over what we eat rather than letting the food control us! Being healthy means taking responsibility for yourself while making peace with the day-to-day realities in life. When you say "No more chocolate for me," you're setting yourself up for failure. Instead, try saying, "I can have as much chocolate as I'd like, but one square will really satisfy me just fine." Now, I admit, this is a delicate balance and can take a long time to master. After years of denying ourselves and then beating ourselves up, it may feel odd to change the pattern. But once you achieve balance, you will free up all that time spent

TONGUE-IN-CHEEK TASTE TEST

Here's an exercise that doesn't require a visit to the gym. Pop a piece of your favorite food in your mouth, and hold it there. What does it taste like? What does the texture feel like? Is it crunchy? Chewy? Gritty? Hot? Cold? Spicy? Sweet? Salty? Notice the flavors and see if you can pull any aromas out of the experience. Exercise the muscles in your mouth and the muscles in your brain to imprint the adventure of really, really tasting delectably delicious foods. Remember, food is one of life's great pleasures, so the lesson here is to learn to truly relish and enjoy it!

thinking and worrying about food for other things—like laughing with your friends and whooping it up for a night on the town!

A healthy, happy, and beautiful woman honors herself and her cravings. When there is something you really, truly want and feel hungry for, have it. Does this mean eating an entire package of cookies at one sitting? *Non, non, cherie!* This means that when you are going to indulge, you do it princess-style. Have a craving for cookies? Then buy the very best cookies you can afford, ones with only the finest-quality ingredients. Put them on one of your sassiest dishes, sit down at the table, and fully enjoy eating them. Had two and are still hungry? Go get two more, and repeat the exercise. Listen to your inner voice! Forget "shoulda, coulda, woulda" and live here, in the moment, right now. Let your taste buds come alive and let yourself engage in the eating experience. As your nutrition guru, I know that if you follow my advice you will be so satisfied that you will not overeat. Why? Because the quality of the eating experience will become so pleasurable that each time you sit down to eat, it will fill up more than just your belly.

The secret to indulging is to balance out your yin with some yang. For instance, I absolutely eat my greens, eat wild Alaskan salmon and organic protein, and drink green tea in place of coffee. But you'd better believe that I love myself some dark chocolate and foie gras. I'll eat my French fries on vacations. And I love a greasy slice of pizza with basil and Parmesan sprinkled on top. I feel fine about these indulgences because for the most part I do what I can to take good care of my body. So there you have it—living proof that it's possible to inject a dose of *la vida loca* into an otherwise healthy body.

AIN'T NO SHAME IN MY GAME

With all this talk about the benefits of indulging now and then, I feel compelled to say a word or two about that evil monster we call guilt. It's all too common—especially for women, and especially in their attitudes toward food. I can't stress enough that a sensual experience does not include guilt. Guilty eating is like carrying around a big bag of bricks—it feels so much better when you just put it down! Bring your food shame out in the open, acknowledge it, and set it free to the universe. So often emotional eating is the symptom, not the root of the problem. The root of emotional eating often stems from the fear of experiencing painful feelings. Rather than face those painful feelings, we eat to make them go away. The process of knowing what you feel and being able to sit with it takes time. When you want to eat and you're not hungry, ask yourself, "What's really going on here?"

Taking the shame out of eating will change your relationship to food in ways you may never have expected. The fear of "I'll never be satisfied" gets replaced with "This is enough for now and I can come back to it later if I want to." Change doesn't happen by force, judgment, criticism, or guilt. Take the first steps toward change by softening the critical voice that runs our life. Isn't it time you reigned as queen over your eating behaviors?

Years ago, I myself worked with a nutritionist while training for the New York City marathon. I had to keep strict food diaries and bring them to her office. I was as honest as I could be (well, I couldn't list *every* martini!) and managed to scribble down my chocolate indulgences. She glared at me over her glasses and circled everything "bad" with a fat red marker. I stared back at her hard and said, "I'm trying to develop a healthy relationship with chocolate here! If I keep it in my house, it's no longer a forbidden food." She said smugly, "There's no such thing as having a healthy relationship with chocolate." I decided to follow my own inner-goddess instincts instead. Who do you think still has chocolate in her cupboard and takes great delight in two squares a few nights a week?

ONE BITE AT A TIME

You may wonder, "Why does everything have to feel so black-and-white for me? I feel like a failure if I don't follow a program 100 percent of the time." I'm here to tell you that the path to food enlightenment starts with one bite at a time. Know that it isn't about perfection but about progress. It isn't about eating perfectly but about feeling comfortable and empowered about your choices. It isn't about being too hard on yourself but about letting go and stretching those personal boundaries. In a nutshell, it's so easy to feel guilty about what we've eaten or should have eaten, but if we spend our time wishing and hoping and yearning, we can't be present in the moment of now.

I've said it before and I'll say it again: Only *you* know what is best for you. Throw away your diet books and wipe the slate clean. Learn to trust your own judgment and check in with yourself. We don't need other people to define our hungers and appetites. We inherently *know* what our bodies need, and we honor ourselves. We create our own rules; we do not need others to tell us what to do—except, of course, when we need a little reminding that eating cookies now and then is a very good thing.

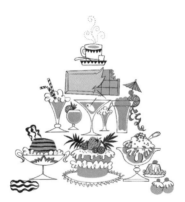

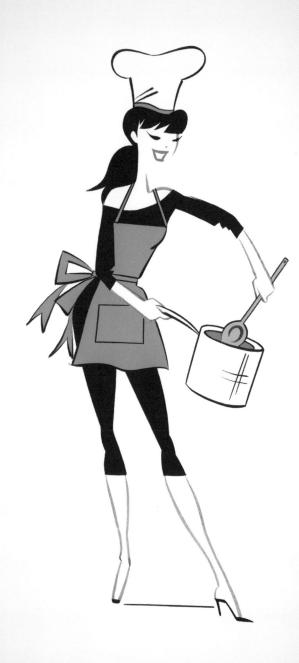

chapter 2

Eating GORGEOUS

One cannot think well, love well, sleep well, if one has not dined well.
–Virginia Woolf

Sure, we'd all like to whip up gorgeously balanced meals at home every day of the week. But in this day and age, it's not so simple. Living the high-octane lives we do, it's nearly impossible to prepare three square meals a day—let alone one. We log long hours at demanding careers, we enjoy bustling social lives, and many of us live in tiny apartments with closet-size kitchens. It's no wonder that most of us spend far more time eating out than we do cooking.

As you may have learned the hard way, eating out while trying to be healthy and/or lose weight can be a bit of a challenge. Many restaurants serve giant-size portions, and it's difficult to know exactly what went into the meal. So in this chapter I'm going to dish on how to eat right while eating out. And to top it off, I'm going to give you some tips on easy, healthy, and delicious meals to make at home. Later on in the book you'll learn how to cook in the bedroom, but for now this sexy swami is going to be your guru in the restaurant and the kitchen! I'm going to guide you through the maze of food options so you can eat gorgeously whether you are eating at home or on the fly. And if you are a novice cook, I'll give you some simple ways to get started in the kitchen. We'll also talk about what to order on a date (there's more on the subject in Chapter 4, "Gorgeous in Bed"), and I'll finish up with a few words about the beauty of juicing. So put down the Bisquick, pick up the buckwheat, and let's get cooking!

FOOD FOR THOUGHT

Before we go any further, it's imperative that we educate ourselves about food's beneficial properties.

The best foods for us to eat are the ones that are minimally processed—by this I mean foods that don't have additives and aren't heavily packaged. You know, fresh fruits, veggies, whole grains, and proteins. Whole foods are richer in nutrition and contain more vitamins and minerals than their processed counterparts. The body is genetically equipped to break down the foods that it can recognize, as opposed to processed foods, which are much

THE PYRAMID SCHEME

Americans have long considered the Food Guide Pyramid the gold standard for nutritious eating. If that's the case, why is obesity reaching epidemic proportions in North America? Could it be that there is a connection between special-interest groups and the recommendations made? As of 2006, the pyramid (which looks more like a triangle with colored stripes) has a foundation consisting of whole-grain bread, rice, cereal, crackers, and pasta; dark green and orange veggies, beans, and peas are listed next; fresh, frozen, canned, or dried fruit after that; milk and dairy next, followed by a little bit of protein and legumes; and oils are hidden underneath the base. It concerns me that with the exception of brown rice, all the so-called grains listed are processed. There is no differentiation between healthy and unhealthy fats, and no differentiation between sugary dried fruits and low-sugar fresh fruits. Like the pyramid before it, the new pyramid continues to contribute to the fattening of America, since it still advocates a diet based on starches without differentiating between good starches and bad starches. To make matters worse, most people don't heed the half-cup servings listed. If I were to redo the pyramid, I'd put vegetables and fruits at the base, protein and legumes as the second tier, unprocessed grains as the third tier, healthy fats as the fourth tier, and processed carbs and sugars in the little triangle at the top.

harder for the body to digest and assimilate. Below you'll find a comprehensive list of foods (protein; carbohydrates, including fruits and vegetables; fats, and dairy) that build an excellent foundation to a healthy diet. I've broken the foods down by type and offered a few suggestions for easy prep. Incorporating these foods will leave you feeling guilt-free and gorgeous. And if you buy organic versions of these foods whenever you can, you'll reap even more health benefits. Don't worry if you can't incorporate all these foodstuffs into your diet; every little thing you do will make a *big* difference.

Protein Power

Looking to fuel your muscles, control your appetite, and stay energized and focused all day long? Look no further than your friend protein. Protein is the ultimate nutritional building block. Our bodies recognize protein as an essential nutrient and can't function without it. Recently we've seen a lot of debate about how much protein we really require. Regardless of the exact measurements, we need to eat meat or other forms of protein to get by in life. When we were hunter-gatherers, we ate a high-protein diet. Why do you think we have incisor teeth?

One of the many beauties of protein is that it shuts off the hunger mechanism in the hypothalamus, in the brain. Starches and carbohydrates don't have the same effect, which is why we can down an entire box of cookies or bowl of cooked pasta and not feel as satisfied. So when you sit down to a meal, always eat the protein portion first.

There are lots of different forms of proteins. Let's look at the nutritional content as a good-better-best scenario. Good is getting any sort of protein—like meat, fish, or chicken—regularly at meals. Better is eating free-range and/or organic protein; certified organic meats or fish are those that have not been administered any hormones or antibiotics, and they have usually eaten a vegetarian diet including corn and soy. Best is to eat grass-fed meats; these are the crème de la crème—raised as nature intended, on natural grass. Grass-fed animals have a leaner body composition than regular farm animals, and their flesh contains more omega-3 fats than fish does. In an era when many fish are contaminated with mercury, this is an excellent option for healthy fats. (See Chapter 7, "Gorgeous Questions and Answers," for more on this subject.) If organic or grass-fed animals are not available or are not in your budget, do the best you can and at least be consistent with your protein intake at meals. Most adults need about three to five ounces of protein per meal.

Primo Proteins

- *Beef.* Make sure your cuts are lean!
- *Buffalo.* It sounds funky, but it's a leaner alternative to beef and contains more protein. Don't knock it till you try it! Buffalo also contains omega-3s.
- *Chicken and turkey.* Lean, mean, and a great source of protein.
- *Fish.* Wild Alaskan salmon has a low mercury content, as do sardines and Alaskan halibut. You can order wild salmon from Vital Choice (vitalchoice.com). Canned salmon is also an excellent source of protein. All fish has some mercury, so eat it judiciously. Steer clear of tuna and swordfish, which the EPA warns against due to their high mercury content.
- *Lamb.* This is a terrific choice for people who have a lot of food allergies.
- *Ostrich.* Same as buffalo—give it a whirl! Buffalo and ostrich should be called the "other red meats."
- *Whey protein.* Remember Miss Muffet on her tuffet, eating her curds and whey? Whey protein is derived from lactose, yet it is virtually lactose-free. It is a great way to incorporate protein into the diet, and it makes a great addition to fruit smoothies, yogurt, and oatmeal.
- *Whole eggs.* Eat both the yolk and the white. The yolk contains more protein than the white, as well as lecithin and choline, which help the liver break down and metabolize cholesterol. Don't believe the hype about eggs raising your cholesterol level; it simply isn't true!
- *All other game meats: pheasant, duck, venison.* Naturally free-range and rich in nutrition, these meats are often available at specialty food stores and online. Venison also contains omega-3s.

Any of the proteins above will do you justice when prepared in a healthful way. Steamed (in the case of fish), roasted, broiled, and grilled are the best way to eat proteins, whether at home or in a restaurant. I like to keep things super simple in the food-preparation department. Here are some general guidelines to healthful (and delicious) prep:

Eggs: Gently boil for 10 minutes. They will be just cooked, but not over-cooked. Hard-boiled eggs are highly portable and make an excellent snack or meal. Boil a dozen at the beginning of the week so they'll be ready to grab and eat!

Beef and Lamb: Good-quality fresh meats often need minimal flavoring; just a little sea salt and pepper will do. If you want to take your taste buds to a new level, finely chop 1 tablespoon of fresh rosemary and combine with 1 crushed garlic clove and 2 teaspoons of olive oil. Brush on top of the meat and bake for 15–20 minutes at 350 degrees F for an incredibly zesty taste.

Chicken: If you roast a whole chicken, simply salt and pepper the outside and inside of the bird. Brush melted butter on top of the bird so it browns in the oven. Bake at 350 degrees F for 1 hour, or until the juices run clear. Feel free to stuff herbs like fresh thyme and rosemary in the center of the bird for extra flavor. For chicken breasts, simply brush on store-bought pesto sauce, sun-dried tomato pesto, or even tomato sauce with fresh Parmesan for a healthier version of homemade chicken Parmesan. Bake for 15 minutes at 350 degrees F.

Fish: Good-quality fish doesn't have to be bland. Brush olive oil, lemon juice, sea salt, and pepper on top and bake for 12–15 minutes at 250 degrees. I also love to top fish with salsa, pesto, sun-dried tomato pesto sauce, or a mixture of pureed olives, sun-dried tomatoes, and fresh garlic. Try it and see what suits you best! Fresh herbs like dill and rosemary also make fish pop.

Turkey: I love to buy premade turkey burgers. They take 12–15 minutes to cook in the oven, at 350 degrees F. I also love to buy organic turkey deli slices. I roll them up with guacamole or mustard for a yummy snack.

Whey Protein Powder: You can stir whey into oatmeal or yogurt for an extra protein kick, or make yourself a protein smoothie: Take 1 scoop of whey protein powder and combine in a blender with 1 cup water, 1 cup frozen berries or a banana, 1 tablespoon natural peanut butter, 2 tablespoons ground flaxseeds, and a dash of cinnamon. Blend with ice. *Bon appétit!*

PEST-ASIDES: SHOPPERS' GUIDE

We all know it's best to eat organic. But sometimes organic produce isn't available or is out of our price range. If you have to pick and choose which fruits and veggies to eat organically, refer to the list below to find out which are most contaminated and which are safest. The Environmental Working Group compiled this list. Check out their Web site at www.foodnews.org.

12 Most-Contaminated Fruits and Vegetables (Buy These Organic):

Apples
Bell Peppers
Celery
Cherries
Imported Grapes
Nectarines
Peaches
Pears
Potatoes
Red Raspberries
Spinach
Strawberries

12 Least-Contaminated Fruits and Vegetables:

Asparagus
Avocados
Bananas
Broccoli
Cauliflower
Corn (sweet)
Kiwi
Mangoes
Onions
Papaya
Peas (sweet)
Pineapples

What about washing? you may ask. Well, while washing fruits and vegetables will reduce pesticide residues, it can't wash away all of the contamination. Many pesticides are absorbed by the plant and simply can't be removed. Other pesticides are created to adhere to the surface of the produce and stubbornly stick regardless of a good scrub. Peeling rids produce of exterior pesticides, but you lose all of the nutrients in the skin. Your best option is to eat organically as much as you can and always wash your fruits and veggies.

Sexy Starches: Carbohydrates

The carb debate is the hottest one in history. Back in the day (the 1980s) the high-carb diet was considered the ultimate in healthy eating. The 1990s brought on the low-carb trend. Today, we're somewhere in the middle. Which suits me fine, seeing as I'm all about moderation.

The reason carbohydrates are such a hot topic is because they can truly have the greatest impact on our weight. Carbohydrates get broken down into sugars before they are absorbed into the bloodstream. That's why it's best to choose high-fiber carbs to slow down the rate at which they are soaked up. Like protein, carbohydrates provide essential nutrients, though only in their unrefined form. I wish I could say cupcakes and cookies were part of our unrefined evolutionary foods, but such is not the case! Bread never grew on trees for that matter, either. So if cake and bread are out (that was so five minutes ago), which starches are good for you? Here's the skinny on the best ones; note that a half cup cooked is a serving size:

- *Barley.* This is a whole grain that is rich in fiber and selenium, normalizing your digestion and your blood sugar.

- *Beans and legumes.* These are high in fiber and are released into the bloodstream at a slow, gradual rate. They'll stabilize your blood sugar and control your appetite for hours after you've eaten, and they have only a minimal impact on your blood sugar.

- *Brown rice.* Loaded with B vitamins, easy to digest, and considered by Eastern medicine to be the most perfectly balanced food, this dietary staple is for you! Make a big pot of it early in the week and reheat portions for dinner.

- *Corn.* Corn is a sugary starch, but it does have health benefits. It is rich in lysine and can help combat cold sores and herpes. Try to buy corn organically whenever possible; a lot of corn is genetically modified and, as a result, has the potential to weaken our immune systems. Also noteworthy is the fact that corn can be difficult to digest, and you may see it leave your body the same form it came in. Ewwww!

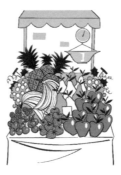

- *Fresh fruits.* Fruits have fiber and anticancer nutrients and make life sweet. You can buy fresh or frozen ones, but beware of canned fruits and fruit juices, which are high in sugar and less beneficial to your health. Dried fruits are loaded with sugar (even without added sugar), and most people eat too much of them, so use them sparingly. Think of them as candy. Berries, pears, and apples contain the least sugar, and pineapple, papaya, mangoes, and bananas have the most.

- *Sweet potatoes.* Lower in sugar than white potatoes, these are a super food that will give you tons of energy. These are chock-full of beta-carotene and potassium and will keep your skin beautiful and improve your immune function.

- *Vegetables.* Dark green, leafy vegetables reign as queen of the greens, ranking highest in nutritional content, but any and all vegetables will do your body good! Organic and fresh are best, and organic frozen ones also make a good choice. Fresh vegetable juices are advantageous; read further on in this chapter to find out more. Skip the canned veggies, since they are probably devoid of nutrients.

- *Winter squash.* These are sweet and fibrous and will keep you full for hours! They're loaded with beta-carotene, which will help fight colds and flus in the winter.

- *Other whole grains, such as buckwheat, quinoa, amaranth, and millet.* These grains have a small amount of protein and have been around for centuries. If everyone ate these more regularly, we'd all be in great shape! Worthy of a girl's respect—even the morning after.

As with protein, it's a cinch to prepare these delicious starches. Cooking whole grains is no great mystery; the simplicity is in the snappiness of it all. Which means you can spend more time getting ready for your date and less time sweating over the steam tray! Here's how:

- *Beans and Legumes:* Don't kill yourself trying to cook them from scratch. Buy the canned versions instead; this is one foodstuff in which the nutrient content will still be retained. Finely chop a sweet onion and sauté it in a skillet with olive oil until it becomes translucent. Then add a can of rinsed beans with a dash each of sea salt, onion powder, and garlic powder. Heat for 5–10 minutes on medium-high, or until bubbly. Sprinkle with cheese if you like, or serve with brown rice for a complete protein.
- *Brown Rice, Barley, and All Other Grains:* Instead of boiling them in water, use chicken broth. Use about four times the amount of fluid as of grains. So if you're cooking ½ cup of brown rice, add in 2 cups of chicken broth. Bring grains and broth to a boil in a pot, reduce the heat to medium, and simmer for 30–45 minutes, or until all the liquid is absorbed.
- *Corn:* Corn on the cob is not only one of the great pleasures of summer, but it's a breeze to prepare. Shuck the corn and pull off all the strands of corn silk. Boil a large pot of water, drop the corn in, and cook for 8 minutes. Pull the corn out and serve fresh, or drizzled with some melted butter and sea salt.
- *Fruits:* Fresh or frozen are best; canned fruits are higher in sugar and rate lower on the nutritional scale. Eat them raw or cook them in a little butter for a sumptuous dessert.
- *Sweet Potatoes:* It doesn't get any easier than this. Preheat the oven to 350 degrees F. Put a piece of aluminum foil on an oven rack in the middle of the oven. Wash the potato with water and a vegetable brush, pat dry with a paper towel, and poke holes into the potato with a fork. Place atop the aluminum foil and bake for 1 hour, turning once midway through the cooking. To serve, cut the sweet potato in half lengthwise and drizzle with olive oil and a splash of sea salt. You can also eat

leftovers with your eggs in the morning, or scoop out the insides and make mashed sweet potatoes.

- *Vegetables:* Heat up a skillet, add in a little olive oil or toasted sesame oil, and sauté them until al dente. Sprinkle with a dash of sea salt and fresh-squeezed lemon juice. For heartier greens such as kale, you will need to tenderize them first by boiling for 3 minutes in water; then sauté. Start simple with spinach leaves or broccoli to build your confidence. You can also try roasting vegetables by tossing chopped vegetables with 1–2 tablespoons of olive oil and $\frac{1}{2}$ teaspoon of sea salt. Cook for 45–60 minutes at 350 degrees F, turning once. This technique does wonders for carrots, Brussels sprouts, fennel, beets, tomatoes, eggplants, asparagus, and countless other vegetables. When they are done, you can sprinkle on freshly grated Parmesan while they're still hot for extra flavor. Use them as a side dish or add them to salads.

GM UH-OHS!

GMOs (genetically modified organisms) made their mark on our foods in 1995. Despite the fact that they have not been approved as safe for human consumption, GMOs appear in 70 percent of processed foods. Unlike the U.S. Food and Drug Administration (FDA), the European Union, Japan, and other nations require labels on GM foods so consumers know what they are buying. Multiple research studies have found evidence that GM foods can pose serious health risks, including damaging the stomach lining and causing antibiotic resistance in humans.

Genetically modified foods are not tested, regulated, or required to be labeled. Soybeans, corn, canola (rapeseed), and cotton are the most widely grown GMO crops. Almost all of these crops are either "insect resistant" or "herbicide tolerant." The list also includes peppers, peanuts, potatoes, sugar beets, sunflowers, and tomatoes. Most of the foreign proteins being gene-spliced into foods have never been eaten by humans before or tested for their safety. Altering genetic structures in humans and plants that have been around for millions of years is a scientific experiment that we can't afford to have go wrong.

- *Winter Squash:* This sort of squash can be a little trickier to prepare. Acorn squash is the easiest; slice it in half and sprinkle it with a little honey, butter, and cinnamon. Bake face up in a glass pan for 45 minutes at 350 degrees F, or until fork-tender. Serve as a side dish. Butternut squash makes a great winter soup, though you must first bake it, peel it, and then puree it in a blender with some chicken stock. You can also take the easy way out and buy premade butternut squash soup, which is also überhealthy for you.

FABULOUS FATS

Fats are another one of those nutrients that spark great debate among nutritionists and scientists. For decades we've been led to believe that all fat is bad. But contrary to popular belief, the right fats can literally make or break your health! Like starches, choosing the healthful ones will help you control your appetite, stabilize your blood sugar, and actually burn fat. Read on to find out which ones will rock your world! And feel free to sneak a peek at the Glossary to learn more about fats.

- *Coconut oil and fresh coconut.* The poor coconut has been given a bad rap for so many years, for no good reason! Coconut has incredible health properties. It fights viruses and boosts the immune system, helps burn body fat, is easy to digest, and is perfect for high-heat cooking. Although coconut contains saturated fat, it helps lower cholesterol. Knock yourself out, baby!
- *Flaxseeds and flaxseed oil.* About 15 percent of the oils present in flax get converted into heart-healthy omega-3s. The seeds are also high in fiber and contain lignans, which help prevent breast and colon cancer and fight constipation. To get the most nutrition out of them, you must grind the flaxseeds before eating them; otherwise, they'll pass through you whole. Keep them in the freezer and store the oil in the refrigerator so they don't go rancid.
- *Grapeseed oil.* Although grapeseed oil contains omega-6 fats, they do not have the unhealthy ramifications of hydrogenated oils. Instead, grapeseed oil is heroic in its ability to withstand high-heat cooking. Use it for baking or sautéing; it has a light flavor.

- *Olives and olive oil.* These contain omega-9 fats and oleic acid. Oleic acid helps your body absorb the omega-3s found in fish oil and flaxseeds. They sensitize your cells to insulin, making it easier for sugar to get into your cells, and for you to burn fat.
- *Raw nuts and seeds.* These contain omega-3s and omega-9s. Omega-3s help fight heart disease and keep your cholesterol levels healthy. Raw nuts and seeds also contain trace minerals that stabilize your blood sugar and control your appetite.

Fats are the basis for bringing out the flavor in meals; you should incorporate some form of fat in your meals to help you absorb the fat-soluble nutrients. Here are some suggestions:

Coconut Oil and Fresh Coconut: Coconut oil contains saturated fat, which makes it extremely stable for high-heat cooking. Use it for frying, popping corn, or any other high-heat cooking. It adds a light flavor to your food and is wonderful in curry sauces. Fresh coconut makes a naturally sweet and rich addition to trail mixes, oatmeal, yogurt, fresh fruit, and freshly juiced green drinks. And for super-dry skin, massage a little coconut oil into your skin—it is incredibly hydrating.

Flaxseeds and Flaxseed Oil: Ground flaxseeds have a pleasant, nutty flavor and make a crunchy addition to yogurt, oatmeal, salads, soups, smoothies, and, yes, even ice cream! You can add them to baked goods, too. Flaxseed oil is more delicate and should be used only as a salad oil or taken straight up; heating the oil destroys the essential linoleic acid within and causes rancidity, which is quite toxic.

Grapeseed Oil: Grapeseed oil has a relatively high smoke point (about 420 degrees F), so it can be safely used to cook at high temperatures. It's a practical choice for salad dressings, stir-fries, sautéing, pancakes, and baked goods. It has a clean, light taste that has been described as "nutty"; I simply think it tastes neutral.

Olives and Olive Oil: Fresh, juicy olives make a fantastic addition to salads and sandwiches, and atop poultry and fish. Or just keep a bowl handy and snack on them during the day—no assembly required! Olive oil is the foundation of the Mediterranean diet and is great for low- to medium-heat

A WATCHED POT NEVER BOILS...

Many people try to delude themselves into thinking that they can't cook. Let me tell you, if you know how to boil water, you know how to cook. Think of all the things that you can make in boiled water: eggs, rice, soup, noodles, corn, beans, vegetables, and fish, for starters. And here's something else that will rock your world: In the time it takes for you to boil a pot of water and cook yourself some pasta, you can pan-sear a steak and sauté some spinach and still have time to mix up cocktails. Now, that's what I call some snazzy sustenance!

cooking, such as lightly sautéed vegetables or scrambled eggs. Use olive oil as a base for salad dressing, drizzle it over raw or cooked vegetables, or be decadent and dip some bread in it. You can also use it on your dry skin après the shower. Delicious!

Raw Nuts and Seeds: So many uses, so little time! Nuts are crunchy and flavorful and kick the fun of your meal up a notch. Try making your own trail mix with an assortment of nuts and seeds. Use ground pecans or pistachios to bread chicken or fish, instead of bread crumbs. Lightly toast them and toss them in your salads. Or grind the nuts in a food processor to make a nut flour that can be used in baking; see www.scdiet.org for nut-flour-based recipes. Nut butters can be used on celery, cucumbers, or apples, in smoothies, or on toast for a yummy treat. I like mine straight off the spoon!

DAIRY? DARE YE?

What's the deal with dairy, and what role should it play in your diet? The answer really depends on your individual makeup. As adults, most of us feel better when we reduce the amount of milk and cheese we eat. Milk causes gassiness for a lot of people, and can cause some people to produce excess mucus in their sinus cavities and throat. And although a glass of milk does contain 8 grams of protein, it also contains 12 grams of the sort of carbo-hydrates that rapidly break down into sugar in the body.

What about cheese, you ask? Hard cheeses can also cause excess mucus production and can exacerbate yeast infections, because they are naturally high in mold. Cheese is basically a fat with a little bit of protein, so nutritionally speaking it should be used in moderation. The best cheeses for you are organic cottage and ricotta cheeses, goat cheese, feta cheese, sheep's-milk cheese, buffalo-milk cheese, and any raw, unpasteurized cheeses you can find. Goat-, sheep-, and buffalo-milk cheeses are usually better tolerated in people who have allergies or sensitivities to cow's milk. And unpasteurized cheeses are richer in calcium than the more processed brands, since the pasteurization process makes it very difficult for calcium to be absorbed.

So if I'm not advocating a lot of cheese or milk, what's left in the dairy family? Yogurt, of course! Yogurt is rich in probiotics, which are the "good" bacteria present in our intestinal tracts. Healthy people normally have about

DON'T BE A BUMP ON A LOG— KEEP A LOG INSTEAD!

If you've never really believed that food can affect your energy levels and mental acuity, try keeping a food log in which you record how you feel before and after each meal. For instance, how do you feel after eating two slices of pizza? How about after a large salad with protein? Or after a sandwich and a soda? Writing it down will help you eat mindfully and make the connections among food, mood, and energy levels.

Keeping It Real: The Food Log

Treat yourself to a sassy little notebook that is for your eyes only. Write down the following:

1. Track your hunger and fullness on a scale at the beginning and end of each meal (see page 46).

2. Think about your emotions at the time you were eating and write them down.

3. Write down the day and time of your meals; this will enable you to keep track of how frequently you eat. Also make sure to write down what foods you ate. Be as honest as you can; remember, it's just good information for yourself to give you a perspective on how certain foods help or hinder your energy levels.

four pounds of beneficial bacteria in their intestinal tract, and yogurt helps keep that balance intact. Yogurt is low in lactose and very easy to digest, making it no surprise that yogurt has been around for billions of years! Now, here's the catch: to get the most benefit, you must buy the plain kind and sweeten it yourself. A cup of yogurt with the fruit on the bottom has 27 grams of carbs, 26 of which are from sugar. This is far too close to the sugar content in a Snickers bar (my personal favorite), which has 30 grams of sugar! If you thought you were virtuous eating that blueberry yogurt, think twice and make the switch to plain. You can sweeten it with a teaspoon of agave syrup, honey, or maple syrup, as well as fresh fruit, and you'll still have a final product that is much lower in sugar.

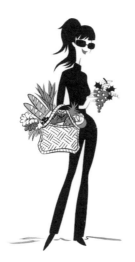

HEY, GOOD LOOKIN', WHATCHA GOT COOKIN'?

Now that you've got the nutritional basics under your belt, it's time to get cooking. Your skill set doesn't matter here. Whether you can't even make toast, you dabble in cooking, or you're a gourmet foodie, you can always tweak your culinary regime to expand your talents and bump up the nutritional content of what you eat. Not to mention that you can also bump up your creative side, as cooking can be an artistic experience (and a sensual one, too)!

Lose Your Kitchen Virginity

What do you need to get started? Like breaking the ice on a first date, you should set aside any cooking fears you may have. After all, what's the worst that can happen? So you burn a little dinner now and then, or you don't like what you taste. Big deal. You throw it out and start over again. You think Jean-Georges or Bobby Flay began by turning out perfect meals every night? All chefs make mistakes; that's how they learn and continue to improve on their craft. I remember the first time I made black beans; I didn't soak them for long enough. They weren't fully cooked (and were therefore difficult to digest), and after eating them my intestines were filled with so much explosive gas I thought I was going to blow a hole through myself! But you live and you learn.

A great icebreaker to your kitchen is to watch cooking shows. *The Barefoot Contessa*, with Ina Garten, and *Nigella Bites*, with Nigella Lawson, are wonderful starters. Rachael Ray busts a move on her show, as does Jamie Oliver on *The Naked Chef*. Seeing other people whipping up simple meals will hopefully inspire you to do the same for yourself, and can encourage you to try new ingredients as well.

You can also stock up on some basic cooking gear that chefs of all levels should have in their kitchens:

A good set of knives	*Reamer*
A set of measuring cups and measuring spoons	*Salt and pepper grinders*
A set of mixing bowls	*Slotted spoon*
Blender	*Spatula*
Can opener	*Timer*
Cutting board	*Tongs*
Frying pan	*Two-quart stockpot*
Garlic press	*Vegetable brush*
Glass baking pan	*Vegetable peeler*
Oven mitts	*Whisk*

Note: When purchasing frying pans, stick to the stainless-steel variety. I'm not a big fan of the nonstick pans, which can release volatile gases like perfluorooctanoic gases (PFOA) into your food when heated over high temperatures. If you insist on cooking with nonstick pans, do not heat them to high temperatures and make sure they are scratch-free, as scratches in the nonstick surface can also release PFOA into your food.

This basic list of kitchen accoutrements will do your kitchen justice for years down the road. Even if you acquire one or two of these items at a time, they will help you rise to the occasion of meal preparation in highfalutin style.

DINING DIVINELY

You now have the 411 on high-quality foods you can eat, and you've even gotten a few pointers on how to prepare them at home. But let's not forget about eating out! It's a fact of life these days that most of our breakfasts and lunches are eaten out on the town, and many of our dinners are, too. Peruse the next paragraphs to find out how to navigate your way through a menu or eat on the go.

QUICK PICKS: EAT AND RUN

So you think you're too busy to squeeze in breakfast, eh? You wake up late after a hard day's night, scrub your face and brush your teeth, slap on some moisturizer, and fly out the door, putting your lipstick on in the elevator. You get to the office and find forty e-mails waiting for you, and both your cell phone and your office line are ringing off the hook. You are a multitasking maniac, are getting progressively crankier, and can't make time for any type of food until 2 P.M., when you're past the point of no return. Whoa, cowgirl—it's time to slow down! You may be a supergirl on the go, but that doesn't mean you can't figure out ways to maximize your morning minutes with some simple nutrition.

Eating breakfast each morning sets you up for success. Like a properly fueled engine, you'll run much more efficiently, with greater energy and mental focus. Eating breakfast starts your inner motor, which helps regulate your weight and your metabolic rate. And trust me, your mood will be better too!

To master morning eating, you need to allow yourself fifteen minutes to prepare and eat it at home or to stop by a deli and pick up something nutritious. If you're going to eat at home, stock your fridge with plain yogurt, fresh or frozen fruit, whey protein powder, steel-cut oats, cottage cheese, eggs, natural peanut butter, and whole-grain bread. If you're going to a deli, you can have the exact same things; the difference is that it's prepared by someone else and costs a little more. See how simple life can be?

Breakfasts of Champions:

- Hard-boiled eggs and steel-cut oats with berries. (Boil up six eggs at a time, and cook steel-cut oats ahead of time in large batches, then reheat single servings for breakfast. Both will keep for one week if refrigerated in an airtight container.)

I'LL HAVE WHAT SHE'S HAVING!

Lunches

- Big bowl of vegetable soup, side salad drizzled with olive oil and vinegar
- Chicken satay skewers with peanut sauce, stir-fried vegetables with bean sprouts
- Turkey or an ostrich burger on a whole-grain bun with veggie slaw
- Create your own salad: mixed greens or spinach, grilled chicken, roasted red peppers, carrots, beets, stuffed grape leaves, and chick-peas tossed with olive oil and vinegar
- Sushi bento box: salmon teriyaki, California roll, cooked spinach

Dinners

- Whole wheat burrito with black beans, rice, vegetables, salsa, guacamole, and chicken
- Sliced duck with wild rice and sautéed spinach
- Grilled chicken, sweet potato, steamed asparagus with lemon juice and olive oil
- Miso soup, salmon-and-avocado sushi roll, eggplant with miso sauce, salad with carrot-ginger dressing
- Filet mignon, baked potato, sautéed broccoli
- Chana saag, lamb biryani, basmati rice, pickled vegetables
- Szechuan chicken, brown rice, steamed snow peas with a shot of soy sauce

- Protein smoothie: 1 scoop whey protein powder, 2 tablespoons ground flaxseeds, 1 tablespoon natural peanut butter, 1 cup frozen berries or a banana, 1 cup water, and a dash of cinnamon. Blend with ice.
- Plain yogurt with ground flaxseeds, fresh fruit, slivered almonds, and agave or maple syrup.
- Vegetable omelet with a side of strawberries.
- Smoked salmon with tomato and avocado slices on whole wheat toast.
- Whole wheat toast with peanut butter alongside sliced cantaloupe.

In the midmorning and midafternoon hours, keep your energy up with some fast, user-friendly snacks. What are the benefits of eating at regular intervals? Eating every three to four hours stokes up your metabolism, gives you strong mental focus, puts your body in a fat-burning mode, keeps sugar cravings at bay, and keeps your blood sugar balanced. A trip to the grocery store once per week will help you prepare these tasty morsels of sheer energy so you can go-go all day long! Pop your snacks in a plastic container so they'll be portable without exploding all over your Prada bag.

Snack Attack:

Hard-boiled eggs

Celery with peanut butter

Turkey slices smeared with avocado and rolled up

Handful of raw nuts

Apple slices with peanut butter

Carrots and hummus

Vegetables and guacamole

Yogurt and fruit

If this list is too Pollyanna for your taste, keep it simple and carry nuts or a piece of fruit with you. No muss, no fuss. Use protein bars for emergency purposes, but don't go overboard, since they usually contain a lot of processed gunk. If you're out of snacks and need to raid the vending machine, stick to pretzels and nuts or cheese and crackers; they're usually the least of the evils. And try to scrounge up some bottled water.

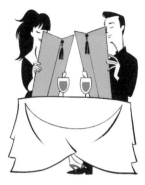

Your Plate or Mine?

I am blessed to live and work in New York City. It is one of the most romantic and fabulous places to date. Restaurants are a dime a dozen, and each one has its own special atmosphere and succulent treasure trove of food. No matter what you're craving—Thai, Japanese, oodles of noodles, or a fat juicy steak—you'll find it here. Upscale restaurants are still catering to the low-carb dieting sector, and even fast-food chains are catching on to the idea that weight loss can sell even when a girl is on the go. But no matter how fabulous the food is, and how much we are enjoying ourselves, one question still remains: What should a Gorgeous Girl eat on a date?

I can't tell you how many times I hear from my clients that they're more stressed about what to order on the date than going on the date itself! If you are trying to eat carefully and the process of eating out seems daunting, take the pressure off yourself by figuring out *what* you want to eat. Feel free to suggest a restaurant that appeals to you ahead of time. Your date will appreciate your initiative, and you'll get to sit back and enjoy yourself. Isn't five minutes of planning worth an evening's peace of mind?

Before we even cover that territory, let me give you the single most important rule for going out in the evenings: Do *not* starve yourself during the day. You *must* eat during the day, especially if you've got a date that night. Eat your breakfast, eat your lunch, and eat one or two snacks in between meals. Nobody likes a party pooper, and if you go all day without meals your blood sugar will plummet, making you a cranky cookie and a very unappealing mood swinger (this is not to be confused with a wild swinger). Whether it's a party or a date, plan ahead of time and make sure you don't neglect yourself during the daytime hours because you're worried about overeating at the big event or trying to keep your tummy flat. If you've taken care of yourself during the day, you will be less hungry by the time nighttime rolls around and less likely to overeat.

GAME-DAY STRATEGIES

The day of your date, keep everything as routine as possible. Don't skip meals or let your hunger get to the point of no return, or your body will attack you warrior-princess-style and you will end up bingeing at dinner to quell your pangs of hunger. You will go to bed with an uncomfortably full stomach, forcing your body to digest during what should be a time of rest. It's just dinner you're going to, not the Last Supper. Grazing and snacking is truly the way to go, rather than saving up all your calories for one giant blowout.

On the following pages are some sample lunch and dinner meal plans that should serve as guideposts for you. Ultimately, you'll need to check in with yourself and decide what on the menu is going to make your taste buds tingle and make the meal that much more enjoyable for you. You should also ask yourself how hungry you truly are when you start to eat; ask again at midmeal to prevent overeating. In a world where stress is abundant and our pleasures are booked within time slots, wouldn't it be wonderful to at least have the knowledge that we're treating ourselves with some level of gentle loving-kindness by giving ourselves what we really need? You're welcome.

If you are going to be consuming alcohol on the date, it is crucial to have food in your stomach beforehand to absorb and metabolize the booze properly. Alcohol initially raises your blood sugar, then lowers it, wreaking havoc on your blood sugar balance, energy levels, sugar cravings, and mood swings. It also loosens up even the best nutritional intentions, making your stomach an unrelenting food whore that just won't quit until it gets paid. Remember, there are peanuts at the bar for a reason, so eat up! (See Chapter 3, "Drinking Gorgeous," for more info on booze.)

Ideally, you'll know ahead of time exactly which restaurant you'll be eating at. That way, you can look up the menu online or have it faxed to you so you can look it over and make sure it appeals to you. (Wouldn't it be a complete disaster to go to an Indian restaurant for the chana saag, only to discover it isn't on the menu?) But what do you do if that option is not available? Here are a few important guidelines:

Eating Right on Date Night

Keep in mind that this info doesn't just apply to date nights. These guidelines work whenever you find yourself in a restaurant.

- Figure out how hungry you are before you start eating. Rate your hunger on a scale of 1 to 10, where a 1 is ravenous and a 10 is overstuffed. Ideally you should start eating at a 2 or 3 and stop somewhere near 5, when you are satisfied. Don't let yourself get too hungry or too full. Somewhere in between is just right.

- Look over the menu and figure out what appeals to you. Do you want something sweet? Salty? Crunchy? Chewy? If you're worried about eating healthfully but just know you won't be truly satisfied until you have the mac and cheese, then just order it and commit to stopping when you're full. Divide the portion in half and see if you are still hungry after the first half is gone. We live in a world where food is abundant; try to remember that you can always come back to it later, *when you are hungry.*

ON THE SIDE, PLEASE

If ordering everything "on the side" is a big thing for you, let me offer a little eating etiquette: It's perfectly okay for you to make specific requests about your meals so that you can get what you want, the way you want it. But please be kind in the process. Remember that your waiter is not your personal butler and, besides, is only human. Be gentle when you ask for sauces on the side or to have an item steamed instead of fried.

And manage your own expectations. If you're in a fast-food chain, don't expect the same high-end service you'd get in a four-star restaurant. Conversely, if you're in a specialty steakhouse, don't expect a large vegetarian selection, lest you be the laughingstock of the table!

- Order a meal that has some protein in it: Lamb, chicken, fish, turkey, ostrich, buffalo, venison, Rock Cornish hen, rabbit, and steak are all excellent choices. When your meal arrives, start by eating the protein first. Protein is the only nutrient that turns off your body's hunger mechanism and will therefore prevent you from overeating.

- Order foods the way you want them cooked. Specify to your waiter whether you'd like something broiled or grilled, if you'd like sauces on the side, or if you'd like substitutions made. Learn to decipher jargon on the menu, or ask the waiter. *Crackling* or *crispy* means something is fried, *grilled* means it is grilled (but usually brushed with oil or marinated beforehand), *sautéed* means that the chef has cooked the food in oil—and usually a fair amount at that—and *poached* means a food is cooked in boiling water or steam. When in doubt, ask.

- If low-carb eating is your bag, then send the bread basket back. Substitute a second vegetable for the starch, and start off with a salad or vegetable-based soup for an appetizer. Did you know that people who eat soup before a meal lose more weight than people who don't? Soups are very filling and low in calories, so you can feel full quickly without eating too much.

- Make sure that you get some fat in your meal as well. Fat will slow down the absorption of foods in your stomach, making you feel fuller longer and turning off your hunger signals, so that ultimately you will end up eating less. Slowing down your digestion will also slow down your absorption of any alcohol you've consumed too quickly, keeping you relaxed enough to enjoy yourself, yet respectable enough to get a second date. The healthiest fat you can find in a restaurant is olive oil. Commercial salad dressings are loaded with thickeners, sugars, and poor-quality oils, so try to stay away from them. Order oil- and vinegar-based dressings, or get a shot of olive oil and vinegar on the side. Feel free to order any salads or appetizers containing avocados, olives, almonds, pecans, sunflower seeds, tahini dressing, or any other nut or seed combo to get a dose of healthy fats as well.

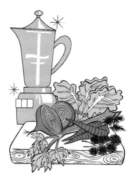

BEING JUICY: VIRGIN SIPS

No chapter on gorgeous eating would be complete without a comprehensive discussion on juicing, which can make you beautiful from the inside out! I have clients that are all over the spectrum when it comes to juicing. Some gals gag at the thought, some want to introduce juices as a snack a few times per week, some want to juice exclusively one day per week for weight-loss purposes, and some want to add it to their daily eating habits. Personally, I love a green juice after working out or to kick a really stubborn cold. It boosts the immune system and gives you energy unlike that from any other food!

One of the greatest benefits of juicing is that it gives you an incredible amount of vitamins and minerals. Most of us do not eat enough fresh vegetables on a daily basis, and juicing can add back some much-needed nutrients into our diets. Juicing is also great for those of us with digestive issues. The fiber and pulp is removed when you juice, enabling nutrients to be easily absorbed across the intestinal wall. This cuts down on the workload required by your digestive system to break down fiber. Green juices also have an anti-inflammatory effect, calm an upset stomach, heal wounds and ulcers, and boost immune function. So if you have a hard time digesting roughage, it's great to add in green vegetable juices on a daily basis.

The downside to juicing is that all too often people consume too much sugar in the process. A good rule of thumb is to never juice more food than you would eat at one sitting. I often see people drinking a large carrot-beet juice combo, which not only has a tremendous amount of sugar but contains up to four or five large carrots and beets apiece. Do you truly eat that many beets and carrots at one sitting? Methinks not. It's also important to remember that the less healthy you are, the harder juicing will be for your system to take. You need to have a baseline of clean eating and adequate protein intake for at least one month before jumping into juicing; otherwise you'll feel pretty sick and will become completely turned off by the whole experience. So ease your way into it. A couple of tips to keep in mind when juicing:

- You don't need your own juicer to get started; visiting a local health-food store that has fresh organic juices will do you right. Costwise it works out to be about the same.
- Mix fruits with fruits and vegetables with vegetables. Fruits are digested more quickly than veggies, so mixing the two together can give you an unwanted case of gas. If you really need to sweeten your juice, add in one beet and/or one carrot.
- Try other enhancers to make your juice taste delicious: lemons, ginger, or shredded coconut make welcome additions. Not only will the coconut taste delectable, but the fat inside will help your body absorb the fat-soluble vitamins in the juice.
- Drink your juice right away, because it is highly perishable.

What is the best mixture of juices? That really depends on your taste buds. Experiment with mixtures of celery, cucumber, spinach, parsley, asparagus, and red-leaf lettuce. Or, if you like to get the pain over with quickly, maximize your potential with minimum volume and do a shot of wheatgrass, my personal favorite. Juicing cilantro is a wonderful mercury chelator, but add this in very gradually, as too much at once can cause headaches. See Chapter 5's cold-and-flu protocol for a delicious juice recipe.

LAST LICKS

Whether you're eating out, cooking in the kitchen, or cooking in the bedroom, have fun and enjoy yourself! Buy organic whenever you can, and try to incorporate some basic home-cooked meals in your regime. If you treat yourself to a sumptuous dinner, balance it out the next day with plenty of green vegetables. At the end of the day, the only person holding you accountable is yourself, and eating gorgeous will help you be your own best friend.

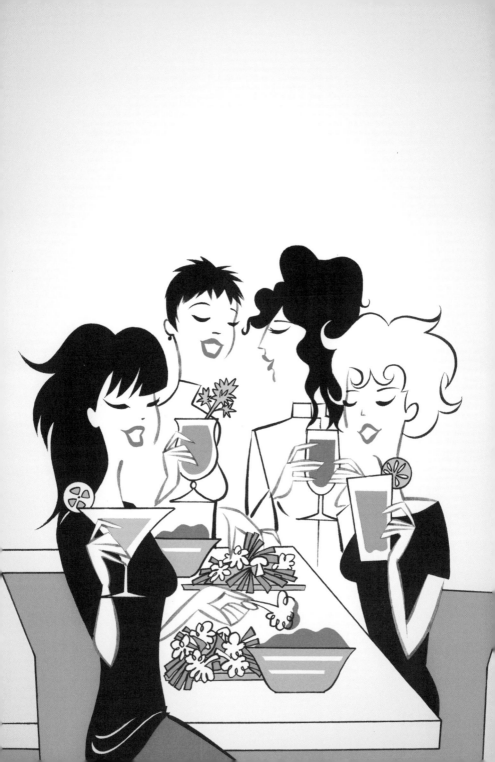

chapter 3

Drinking GORGEOUS

I love to drink martinis,
Two at the very most.
Three, I'm under the table.
Four, I'm under the host!
—Dorothy Parker

Saturday night: You're gussied up, glittering, glamified, and gorgeous. A dash of perfume and you're out the door and on your way to the club, where you'll meet up with your best pals, cozy up to the bar, and order a delicious, frosty cocktail. *Ahhh.* They don't call it a social lubricant for nothing. Alcohol is the perfect party starter—but we all know you can go from glam to slammed in no time at all, with just one glass too many. And while the flight up into inebriation is oh so heavenly, the morning after can be nothing short of a highway to hell. There is not one gal out there who hasn't relied too heavily on liquid courage at one time or another, and at some point, everyone wakes up with a hangover.

When I say everyone, I mean *everyone.* Just because I'm a nutrition-ist doesn't mean that I'm immune to the perils of living it up too large! I, too, have paid the price for having had one too many drinks. I am a social butterfly by nature, and anyone who knows me can tell you that I hate to miss a party. But through the years, I have learned how to dazzle, partake, and par-*tay* without breaking a sweat (or anything else) at a party. And I'm here to tell you how.

Being healthy *and* the belle of the ball is no small feat, mind you. Whatever you pick as your poison (be it a Miller, a Manhattan, or Merlot), do remember that it is just that—a poison—and your responsibility to yourself is to help your body metabolize the poison in the best way possible. If you've had one hangover too many and your mantra has become "Never again!," I'm the maharishi to guide you down the path of alcoholic enlightenment. Follow my advice and you'll be able to have your cocktail and drink it too. I'm going to give you the straight dope on which alcohols do the least damage, how to prevent hangovers, and how to manage them. I've organized the chapter into four sections. Look to "Cruising for a Boozing" to find out how alcohol affects your system. "Don't Do the Crime if You Can't Do the Time" provides tips on what to eat and which supplements to take to prevent hangovers and decrease the toll alcohol can take on your system. The "Short-Term Measures" section puts at your fingertips many ways to prep your body for a big night out. And last but not least, "Relief Is on the Way" outlines all sorts of remedies, in case you didn't do your homework before you got loaded. For you sexily sober babes out there, read on further; there's something here for everyone!

Before we get to the good stuff, no chapter on drinking would be complete without a disclaimer. This chapter is in no way, shape, or form a license to ill! My intent is to provide you with support and rescue remedies for an accidental overdose of hooch, not to empower you to get screaming drunk every night. Gorgeous Girls need to take responsibility for themselves and not act like drunken asses *all* the time. I'm a dietitian, not a magician, and I have vitamins, not a magic wand! So rather than get excited about going out and binge-drinking, let's switch gears a little bit and think about consequence-free, grown-up drinking that will keep you fresh as a daisy *le* morning after.

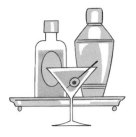

CRUISING FOR A BOOZING: ALCOHOL AND ITS EFFECTS

If you just want to cut to the chase and learn how to get rid of your hangover, skip this section and move right along to "Relief Is on the Way." But once the pounding in your head has subsided, revisit this section to learn about the long-term effects alcohol has on your body.

CANDY IS DANDY, BUT LIQUOR IS QUICKER: HOW YOUR BODY PROCESSES ALCOHOL

Despite the fact that a moderate amount of alcohol has proven health benefits (see Chapter 7, "Gorgeous Questions and Answers"), too much alcohol is toxic. A hangover is a constellation of unpleasant symptoms that occurs eight to sixteen hours after you drink excessive amounts of alcohol. Characterized by headaches, tremors, nausea, diarrhea, dry mouth, soreness, weakness, dizziness, and loss of appetite, a hangover also impairs your vision, cognitive functions, and spatial skills. The reason you feel so lousy after a hard night's drinking could be a combination of dehydration, hormonal changes induced by alcohol, direct toxic effects of alcohol, and inflammation caused by metabolizing alcohol, or it could be a result of impurities in the beverages.

When you drink, your body converts alcohol into toxic by-products. When breaking down these toxic by-products, the liver's Phase I process (see "Love Your Liver," page 54, for more info) produces free radicals, which are like little pinballs that seek electrons from other cells in order to make themselves more stable. If you drink too much, the free radicals are produced in excess, which can harm your liver cells. As they bounce from cell to cell, they can damage your DNA and ultimately make your cells act sick and age at a faster pace. This damage is to blame for the hangover experience.

In addition to making you feel crummy, the free radicals can disrupt normal, everyday cellular activities throughout your body that enable you to function. They can turn good cholesterol bad, cause cataracts, contribute to Alzheimer's disease, and lead to cancer. Damage accumulates over time, injuring the cells' walls and ultimately our DNA. Extensive DNA damage shuts down the mitochondria, or the cell's furnace, causing the cells to die, which fuels the aging process within us. This damage plays out differently for everybody; for some babes it's wrinkled skin, for others it's feeling more tired, and for others it's storing extra body fat.

Love Your Liver

The liver is a girl's best friend. Truly. It has the huge job of metabolizing and removing poisons in the body, whether it be too much alcohol, environmental toxins such as mercury or pesticides, or too much estrogen or medication. It's pistol-whip smart and will tell you right away if it doesn't like something by giving you a royal hangover or a kink in your digestion. When you are out drinking with the girls, it works double-time to keep you sober.

Much like a washing machine, the liver has its cycles: Phase I detoxification and Phase II detoxification. The general purpose of the whole detoxification process is to convert fat-soluble toxins (toxins that dissolve in fats and would therefore be trapped in your body) into water-soluble substances (toxins that dissolve in water and can be excreted from the body). If this does not occur, the toxins cannot be eliminated from the body and will stay inside the fat cells, which can lead to the appearance of cellulite.

In Phase I detoxification, a series of chemical reactions causes the liver to convert toxic chemicals into less harmful chemicals. Enzymes are required for this reaction; grouped together, they are termed the cytochrome P-450 system. Phase II detoxification converts the less harmful substances of Phase I detoxification into water-soluble substances that the body can excrete via the kidneys and bladder. To work efficiently, Phase II detoxification requires certain sulfur-containing amino acids (taurine and cysteine), as well as substances like glutathione, the liver's most potent antioxidant. If the Phase I and II detoxification pathways become overloaded with waste products, there will be a buildup of toxins in the body. Taking medication, eating junk food, and being exposed to environmental pollutants such as gas fumes can all clog up the liver and make it harder for it to run efficiently.

It's Different for Girls: Why Your Cups Runneth Over

A woman's body breaks down alcohol more slowly than a man's does. Because of several physiological differences, you will feel the effects of alcohol more than a man will, even if you are the same size. (This makes us much cheaper dates.) The reason is that we have significantly less dehydrogenase, a liver enzyme that breaks down alcohol. Typically women metabolize one drink per hour, while men metabolize two. Having more than one drink per hour will slow your motor function and coordination. Consume three drinks in an hour and you might be tossing them back up, especially if you've mixed your alcohols (a complete disaster and a guarantee for a hangover the next day).

There is also increasing evidence that women are more susceptible than men to alcohol's damaging effects. Heavy drinking (two or more drinks per day) has been shown to disrupt normal menstrual cycling and reproductive function, putting you at increased risk for infertility, spontaneous abortion, or impaired fetal growth and development.

When a woman drinks, the alcohol in her bloodstream typically reaches a higher level than a man's, even if both are drinking the same amount. This is because women's bodies generally have less water than men's bodies (52 percent for the average woman versus 61 percent for the average man). Because alcohol mixes with body water, a given amount of alcohol is less diluted in a woman's body than in a man's. Women become more impaired by alcohol's effects and are more susceptible to alcohol-related organ damage. Ain't womanhood grand?

And it doesn't stop there. During the days right before you get your period, premenstrual hormonal changes can also make intoxication set in faster. It's also pertinent to know that birth control pills or other medications containing estrogen will slow down the rate at which alcohol is eliminated from your body. Be mindful, too, when combining alcohol with antidepressants. Many people who take Zoloft, Prozac, or other depression-related medications can drink light to moderate amounts of alcohol without serious side effects, or any unusual effects at all. However, it's never advisable to mix alcohol and antidepressants. When there is a noticeable reaction from mixing alcohol with antidepressants, it's often an amplified response to the alcohol, and one drink could end up feeling like two. If you usually feel tired or even a bit depressed after drinking, then you might feel even more so if you're on antidepressants. Alcohol also affects the serotonin levels in your brain by altering production levels. That's why using these two drugs together could produce unexpected and unwanted reactions.

WILL HOOCH GIVE ME A POOCH?

Ladies, I'm afraid I don't have good news. Although alcohol itself doesn't contain any fat, it is metabolized as a fat. The reason is that alcohol is not an efficient fuel, so it actually halts your body's fat-burning process. Protein and carbohydrates contain 4 calories per gram, alcohol contains 7 calories per gram, and fat contains 9 calories per gram. So if you're a gal who likes her liquor, remember that it's easy to gain weight from drinking, because not only is alcohol packed with calories, but it increases your appetite to boot! And when you add in mixers—juice, sugar, and other ingredients—the calories really can add up. Here's a handy breakdown of calories in different types of drinks:

Beer: Nonalcoholic beer actually has the same calories as alcoholic beer: 148 calories in a twelve-ounce serving. If you drink a light beer—like Bud Light—you'll take in only around 99 calories per twelve ounces. But if you drink the heavy ales and porters, you can bet your bottom dollar that the calorie count will shoot up instantaneously.

Wine: Dry wine contains fewer calories than sweeter wine. For example, a glass of dry wine has about 106 calories and a glass of sweet dessert wine a whopping 226. If you drink a glass of wine before dinner, another glass with dinner, and a sweet wine for dessert, you've added more than 400 calories to your meal.

Champagne: You'll be glad to hear that champagne contains the same amount of calories as other dry wines: 106 per glass.

Hard Alcohol: The calories in gin, rum, vodka, and whiskey depend on the proof, which is twice the percentage of alcohol. For example, 90 proof vodka is 45 percent alcohol; 100 proof vodka is 50 percent alcohol. It's easy to guess

WHERE DO YOUR DRINKS WEIGH IN?

I've listed the calorie contents of a mélange of cocktails so you'll know where on the scale your drinks weigh in. Unless otherwise noted, the calories listed for wine are based on a 4-ounce serving and beer servings are 12 ounces. Daiquiris, martinis, and Manhattans are approximately 4 ounces.

Amstel Light beer: *95 calories*

Bloody Mary: *115 calories*

Budweiser: *160 calories*

Champagne, dry: *106 calories*

Chardonnay: *90 calories*

Chocolate martini: *188 calories*

Coors Light beer: *102 calories*

Cosmopolitan: *179 calories*

Dos Equis imported beer: *160 calories*

Eggnog: *305 calories*

Frozen margarita: *246 calories*

Gimlet: *110 calories*

Gin and tonic: *171 calories*

Guinness Extra Stout: *190 calories*

Heineken beer: *160 calories*

Hot toddy: *150 calories* *(per 3 ounces)*

Irish coffee: *159 calories*

Jack Daniel's and Coke: *129 calories*

Kahlúa and cream: *90 calories* *(1.5 ounces)*

Mai tai: *306 calories*

Manhattan: *183 calories*

Martini: *210 calories*

Michelob Ultra: *95 calories*

Miller Genuine Draft: *148 calories*

Miller Light beer: *110 calories*

Mimosa: *137 calories*

Mudslide: *155 calories*

Newcastle Brown Ale: *150 calories*

Pete's Wicked Ale: *174 calories*

Piña colada: *342 calories*

Red Bull with vodka: *210 calories*

Red wine: *90 calories*

Rum and Coke: *240 calories*

Rum and Diet Coke: *133 calories*

Samuel Adams: *145 calories*

Samuel Adams Boston Lager: *160 calories*

Sangria: *115 calories*

Schlitz Light beer: *110 calories*

Screwdriver: *208 calories*

Strawberry daiquiri: *150 calories*

Strawberry margarita: *210 calories*

Whiskey sour: *122 calories*

And the winner of the most calories per drink goes to…the 8-ounce margarita, which clocks in at a whopping 540 calories! Don't go at it alone; grab some friends and some straws and divvy it up!

which has more calories: The higher the proof, the higher the calories. Here's the damage:

- A double shot of 80-proof liquor contains 97 calories

- A double shot of 90-proof liquor contains 110 calories

- A double shot of 100-proof liquor contains 124 calories

Liqueurs: The calorie content of other types of liquor varies greatly. Watch the really sweet stuff. A serving of schnapps has 108 calories, and crème de menthe will set you back 186 calories. Why do you think they're served in shot glasses?

Mixed Drinks: Obviously, the larger the mixed drink, the higher the calorie content. If your favorite watering hole serves 8-ounce pond-sized margaritas, you can easily drink more than 500 calories in one fell swoop (that's without the chips and guacamole). Choose a smaller cocktail, like a cosmopolitan, and you'll take in only about a third of the calories; but keep in mind that a cosmo is still quite sugary.

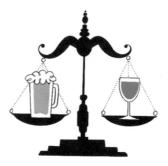

ADDING IT ALL UP

One beer every night adds 1,036 additional calories per week, or fifteen pounds to your stomach per year. Can we say "beer belly," anyone? Three glasses of dry wine a week will cost you 318 calories, or an additional three miles on the treadmill just to walk off the extra calories.

LIQUEFIED AND LOVING IT!

To calculate exactly how many ounces of water you need a day, divide your body weight in half; that's the number of ounces to shoot for. So a 150-pound person would need to drink 75 ounces of water, or nine glasses (8 ounces per glass) of water per day. For every twenty minutes you exercise, you will need to drink an additional 4 to 8 ounces of water. For every caffeinated or alcoholic beverage you consume, you will need to drink another 8 ounces of water, to compensate for their dehydrating effects.

What drinks are the best antidotes for dehydration? The best and most pure is, of course, filtered water. So make your way over to the water-cooler, pronto! If you're not crazy about plain old water, you've got other options. Grab a bottle of seltzer, dilute a shot of pomegranate juice into a glass of water, or chill out with herbal teas. Spice up regular water with slices of lemons, limes, oranges, or cucumbers for a delicious and healthy treat! And don't forget to invest in a good at-home filter to remove impurities such as lead, rust, chlorine, and cryptosporidia from the tap water.

If you're watching your weight, follow these tips:

- Limit your alcohol intake to three drinks per week. From a health and hangover perspective, space them out over the course of a week, rather than binge-drink them all at once.
- Remember that the calories from alcohol add up quickly, and they go straight to the fat in your abdomen; visualize a muffin top hanging over your waistband!
- Most people eat high-calorie snacks when they drink alcohol—a double whammy in terms of weight gain.

Makes club soda with a twist of lemon look all the more angelic, doesn't it? Damn!

DON'T DO THE CRIME IF YOU CAN'T DO THE TIME: LONG-TERM PREVENTION TIPS

That double martini isn't sounding so good anymore, is it? Fear not: Your nutritional fairy godmother is here to dispense some lifestyle tips so you can enjoy a cool cocktail now and then without the nasty hangover.

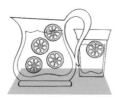

H2Ohhhhhh!

When you're talking about drinking, water is the do-re-mi, the very beginning, the perfect place to start. You know that drinking water is good for you, but did you know that every system in your body depends on water? On average, both men and women need to drink eight to ten 8-ounce glasses of water daily. On average, most adults lose about ten cups of fluid a day through sweating, exhaling, urinating, and bowel movements. Even minor dehydration can cause you to lose concentration and experience headaches, irritability, or fatigue. For you teetotalers out there, and especially for you Boozy Suzies, this section is a must! Read on about the importance of staying hydrated and the health benefits that water can bring into your life.

Why does water do your body good? First and foremost, water makes you gorgeous! Drinking water moisturizes and hydrates your skin from the inside out. It's essential to maintaining elasticity and suppleness, and it helps prevent dryness. Secondly, water is nature's weight-loss tool. Increasing your water consumption prevents you from confusing hunger with thirst. Often, especially in the wee hours of the night, we reach for food when in reality it is water our body needs. Water will also keep your body systems, including your metabolism and digestion, working properly. Last but not least, water puts some pep in your step and keeps you bright-eyed and bushy-tailed. It literally breathes air into your cells, providing the essential energy (and hydration) necessary for exercise, and it comprises a large part of the fluid that lubricates and cushions your joints and muscles. Drinking water before, during, and after exercise can help reduce muscle cramping and premature fatigue.

Best of all, water also curbs hangovers. It helps the body flush toxins, lessening the burden on your kidneys and liver. And, given the fact that alcohol is extremely dehydrating, replacing liquor-induced losses is the ticket to looking and feeling good!

With all the benefits water has to offer, you may ask yourself if too much water is bad for you. Although it rarely happens, there have been some reported cases of people dying from hyperhydration. Drinking too much water can decrease the sodium in your blood to extremely dangerous levels. The average person can process slightly more than a glass of water per hour. So remember, there is a difference between optimizing your hydration and overdoing it.

An Ounce of Prevention Is Worth a Pound of Allure

In the case of hangovers, prevention is even better than the cure. Rather than trying to put a soothing balm on a wicked hangover that just won't quit, let's pull out the big guns and stop that crazy train before it leaves the station!

Eat your greens, beauty queens! Antioxidants can reduce and even repair some of the damage caused by free radicals, as they act like shields of armor to protect the outside (and sometimes the inside) of the cell. The liver uses the vitamins, minerals, and phytonutrients found in vegetables like kale, Brussels sprouts, barley grass, buckwheat, and alfalfa to protect its cells from oxidative damage. And if your liver is functioning optimally at all times, your ability to break down unhealthy compounds will keep you feeling fit and fabulous for a lifetime. *Now* do you see why you've been summoned all these years by a tall, dark, and handsome Jolly Green Giant? He really had your number, Miss Ho Ho Ho!

Incorporating dark green, leafy vegetables into your diet will benefit your body in so many ways. Cleaning up your liver, skin, heart, immune system, and intestines is just the beginning of the health and beauty payoffs:

- *Broccoli, kale, and Brussels sprouts* contain indoles that prevent cancer and glutathione compounds that carry out detoxification reactions. This will enable your liver to remove the toxic alcoholic by-products efficiently and effectively. Kale and Brussels sprouts help the liver perform the job of detoxification, rendering harmful substances like alcohol and tobacco into waste products that the body can eliminate.

• *Barley grass, buckwheat, and alfalfa:* Barley grass and alfalfa are great sources of protein and contain a wide array of vitamins, minerals, and enzymes that are crucial for maintaining health. Alfalfa contains chlorophyll, which protects against environmental carcinogens. Chlorophyll binds to toxins and deactivates them by preventing them from binding to DNA and cellular receptors, decreasing the cellular damage caused by drinking. Buckwheat contains rutin and quercetin, two antioxidants that offer cellular protection against oxidative damage; they also protect the body and the liver from alcohol-induced damage. Barley grass is great for treating an upset stomach, diarrhea, gastritis, and inflammatory bowel conditions, all of which can be exacerbated by alcohol.

• Long-term use of *DMAE* supplements (200 mg per day) can eliminate many of the symptoms of hangovers. DMAE is most effective when taken in the morning on an empty stomach.

• *Zinc* (25–50 mg per day) ensures that the enzyme that detoxifies hangover-causing acetaldehyde is at optimal levels.

The cruciferous creatures listed above are the goddesses of the greens in terms of supporting liver function. But I also ask you to leave room on your plates for beets, which support gallbladder function and facilitate digestion; all other leafy green vegetables, which give you the most bang for your nutritional buck; and shots of wheatgrass, which are rich in chlorophyll, neutralize toxins in the body, and purify the liver.

SHORT-TERM MEASURES FOR CURTAILING THOSE POST-PARTY HANGOVERS

There are tons of little things you can do to prevent a nasty hangover before you go out. Forget about being naughty for a moment and think about being nice to your body—in a few simple steps you can put a stop to something before it starts. Long-term prevention is your hangover-free foundation; in this section, I'm going to reveal ways you can accessorize your hangover-free house!

Dine While You Wine

First and foremost, babes who love their booze must remember that drinking on an empty stomach is a big no-no. Let's look to our European mentors for a little inspiration here. I've been blessed in life to have traveled to some of the most fabulous places in Europe: the Pyrenees in Spain and France, islands off the coast of Sicily, the French Riviera, and, of course, Paris, where I spent an afternoon spying on Quentin Tarantino, who sat one table away from me at Les Deux Magots.

While on holiday, my treat to myself is to transition from afternoon into evening with a glass of wine or beer. Now, I was brought up in a Jewish household where you never drank but you always ate, so for me it is sheer bliss knowing that before the European server even comes to take your drink order, adorable little *nosherai* magically appear on the table—petite bowls of olives, potato chips, smoked nuts, and tiny vegetable sticks with even tinier bowls of tangy dip are just some of the scrumptious goodies I have nibbled on between sips of my drink. The whole system is just perfect for me; in Europe, alcohol is almost always enjoyed with food. It's not just a means to the end of getting plastered. So I advise all my clients to take a tip from our European friends: While you can certainly get a great buzz eating food with your drink, having food in your stomach all the while is a great way to offset a hangover the next day.

Punch Drunk

Before I went to college, my brothers warned me to stick to beer at frat parties. There's no way to know what's in those mixed punches and, therefore, no way to know how much alcohol you're swilling. Imagine thinking that you're drinking vodka when you've really been drinking grain alcohol—ouch! As a general rule, hangovers are more common with distilled, stronger alcoholic drinks and less so with red wine, champagne, white wine, and beer. You're a lot less likely to get hangovers if you follow a few simple rules:

- Skip the sugary daiquiris, margaritas, and cosmopolitans. Sugar is a speedboat in the cellular ocean that carries the effects of alcohol full speed ahead! Not only that, but the sweet taste makes them go down much faster. Raise your hand if green apple martinis have gotten you seriously bombed at one point or another.

- Check in with yourself. If you want to avoid getting too tipsy too quickly, then order a water or soda with lime between cocktails. That way you'll stay hydrated and keep a low-level buzz going for longer. If you can't bear to order a water, at least alternate concentrated drinks with diluted ones. Instead of two straight martinis, have one vodka martini and one mixed drink that combines vodka, club soda, and a shot of cranberry juice.

- Put some hair on your chest and learn to drink hard alcohol with as few mixers as possible. I'm not saying you should slam down shots, but sipping whiskey on the rocks or vodka neat will do you justice. Can't do it, you say? Soda water (that is, club soda or flavored club soda) will make most drinks pretty palatable. Not only will you save yourself a lot of calories, but you'll avoid the unknown sugars in the mixers—and Lord knows what other alcohols that have been thrown in.

- Say no to caffeine. Think it's going to help keep you energized and fresh? Think again. Caffeine suppresses ADH (antidiuretic hormone), which makes you pee more, ultimately dehydrating you. Yes, it will keep you going while you're out on the town but, man, you'll feel it the next day. And if you're the type of gal who can't drink coffee at night because it interferes with your sleep, then you'll be singing the same old song after another night of lousy sleep.

- Finish drinking early enough to let your body metabolize as much alcohol as possible before going to bed. Your body's functions slow down when you sleep, which slows down the rate at which you eliminate the alcohol from your body. Staying up a little longer also gives you time to drink two or three glasses of water before going to bed. Trust me, even if you lose an hour or two of sleep by staying awake to sober up, you'll feel so much better than if you pass out cold.

- Try to get enough rest to enable your body to burn off the alcohol. Generally you burn off about two-thirds of a drink per hour; this rate may slow down while you're sleeping. So give yourself extra time to sleep in and rest the next day; a day-after-the-disco nap will do you good!

- If you take a painkiller to offset a potential headache, skip the acetaminophen (found in Tylenol) and head for something ibuprofen-based (like Advil). The ingredients in Tylenol are harder on the liver, which is already overworked, and cause greater toxicity when mixed with alcohol.

Nutritious and Delicious

In today's health-conscious age, we all want to do just a little better for ourselves without going completely overboard. Did you know that by giving your cocktails a makeover you are doing something healthy for yourself? Small changes make a big difference, even if they're encased in spirits!

Instead Of...	Try...
Apple martini	Green tea martini
Cosmopolitan	Pomegranate martini
Vodka on the rocks	Citron vodka with raspberry club soda
Red Bull with vodka	Diet Vanilla Coke with vanilla vodka
Gin martini	Gimlet
Gin and tonic	Gin and Diet Sprite
Dark ale	Light beer

THE PECKING ORDER OF DRINKING

Is the saying "Beer before liquor, never sicker; liquor before beer, never fear" physiologically accurate? No, my darlings. It's just this simple: Mixing different types of alcohol is generally a bad idea. It's possible that the *reasoning* behind the proverb is that it's easier on your body to absorb weaker alcoholic drinks, like beer, later in the evening. But any piece of advice regarding alcohol consumption that contains the line "never fear" is obviously pretty suspect.

HALT THE HANGOVER

If you want to drink alcohol without suffering from a hangover the next day, consider taking cysteine (200 mg) plus vitamin C (600 mg) prior to drinking, with each drink, and once again right after you finish drinking. Many drinkers find that this strategy results in a hangover-free following day. (All the extra water you must drink when taking these pills certainly doesn't hurt, either!)

- Some people replace regular cysteine in this combination with N-acetyl cysteine (NAC), although this form may be slightly less effective.

- The addition of vitamin B_6 (50 mg) to this regime further enhances its effectiveness for preventing hangovers.

- Also take 150 mg of milk thistle twice per day, with 250 mg of schisandra.

- Take 2 evening primrose oil capsules (1,000 mg each) before heading out on the town.

- DMAE has also been shown to help prevent hangovers: take 200 mg per day.

RELIEF IS ON THE WAY

Uh-oh! If you're reading this section, you're probably suffering from a hangover and need a virtual life preserver to bring you to dry land! This section lists restorative antitoxins that will offer you some cushioning to the blow your poor body has been dealt. Once you have them in your medicine cabinet, you'll never know how you lived without them all this time.

VITAMINS: RESCUE REMEDIES AND HANGOVER HELPERS

The right supplements can do wonders in preventing and relieving hangovers. And if you think you're above it all just because you've built up a carefully crafted tolerance, stop right there in your high-heeled tracks. Even alcoholics get hangovers—why do you think they need to keep drinking? Now, my darlings, I'm going to teach you about the vitamin cocktail that will remedy what ails you. Not only should you take these supplements after overindulging, but it's great to take them every day for daily detoxing. If you suffer from PMS, this regime will help your symptoms because it supports liver function. Hooray! The nutrients listed below provide the vitamins and compounds necessary to replace the damaged enzymes, help get your system back on track, and keep the Krebs and glycolytic energy cycles going. The result? You can move on with your life and get on with your day.

Evening Primrose Oil: An essential fatty acid that improves circulation, helps regulate inflammation, and relieves pain. There is some evidence to suggest that this herb may lessen cravings for alcohol. The main active ingredient of evening primrose oil is gamma-linoleic acid (GLA), an omega-6 fatty acid that can also be found in borage and black currant oils. *Dosage:* 1,000–2,000 mg per day.

NAC (N-Acetyl Cysteine): NAC is an altered form of the amino acid cysteine, which is commonly found in food and synthesized by the body. NAC helps the body synthesize glutathione, an important antioxidant. In animals, the antioxidant activity of NAC protects the liver from the effects of exposure to several toxic chemicals. In humans, NAC helps drive out the toxins acquired from booze and tobacco smoke. *Dosage:* 1,000–1,500 mg per day.

Vitamin B_6 and Lipoic Acid: There are several other nutrients that may work synergistically with cysteine and vitamin C. Vitamin B_6 and lipoic acid are key sulfur-containing nutrients that may be depleted by alcohol and may help with acetaldehyde detoxification. Vitamin B_6 has been proven to further enhance the ability of the combination of cysteine plus vitamin C to prevent hangovers. *Dosage:* 300 mg per day of B_6; 300 mg per day of lipoic acid.

Vitamins C and E: Research shows that vitamins C and E and the amino acid cysteine act as an antioxidant force to counter acetaldehyde-produced free radicals, helping to protect against long-term damage. *Dosage:* 500–1,000 mg per day of vitamin C; 400 IU of vitamin E—try to find a food-based supplement for these.

Magnesium: Many of the symptoms of hangovers are believed to come from the magnesium depletion that occurs when you drink alcohol. Supplementing your diet with additional magnesium helps counteract hangover symptoms that stem from a lack of magnesium. *Dosage:* 400 mg per day of magnesium glycinate (this is a highly absorbable form of magnesium).

DMAE: A clinical study found that a derivative of choline named dimethyl-aminoethanol (DMAE), when taken for at least six weeks, resulted in subjects

HAIR OF THE DOG?

Although the phrase "the hair of the dog that bit you" originally referred quite literally to a cure for dog bites, people often use the phrase when having an "eye-opener" the morning after a big night out drinking. Why? you ask. To try to alleviate the symptoms of a hangover by drinking more alcohol! If you're looking for a convenient excuse to crack open a can of Schlitz at 10 A.M. on a Sunday, then go for it! But as your Venus de No-No, I must warn you that it's not such a great idea, since your body has not finished metabolizing all the alcohol from the night before. Let's take a quick look at some of the supposed morning-after "remedies," just for fun:

Bloody Mary

Mimosa

Black Velvet (a mix of champagne and flat Guinness)

Tomato juice and beer (Hemingway's tonic)

A "red-eye": whiskey, coffee, Tabasco sauce, a raw egg, pepper, and orange juice blended together

Raw eggs

Hot coffee

Lots of ice-cold Coke, ginger ale, or Gatorade

A greasy breakfast

The Greeks are my heroes: They munched on cabbage! Fantastic liver support.

LEMON SOUR POWER

Annemarie Colbin, a holistic nutritionist and a wonderful mentor, swears by Mother Celestina's Tea for headaches associated with stress on the liver. Juice half an organic lemon, reserving juice in a cup. Slice the rind from the juiced half in quarters and simmer in 1¼ cups of boiling water covered, for 10 minutes. Strain the water into the cup with the juice. If juice is too tart, add ½ teaspoon of honey. Drink hot.

being free of the headaches and irritability that normally occur with hangovers. *Dosage:* 200 mg per day.

MSM: Methylsulfonylmethane (MSM) is a good source of sulfur, which may counteract the ability of acetaldehyde to initiate hangovers. This therapy has not yet been tested in clinical trials, but many of my "research subjects" claim that it rapidly (within twenty minutes) alleviates the symptoms of hangovers. *Dosage:* 1,000–3,000 mg per day.

Zinc: As mentioned previously, the enzyme acetaldehyde dehydrogenase stimulates the conversion of hangover-causing acetaldehyde (derived from alcoholic drinks) into acetic acid (used for energy production). Ensuring that you obtain plenty of zinc should theoretically maximize the availability of this enzyme to divert acetaldehyde toward energy production rather than permitting acetaldehyde to exert its toxic effects, which result in hangovers. *Dosage:* 25–50 mg per day.

Silymarin (milk thistle): Milk thistle is a potent antioxidant that has been shown to protect the liver and enhance its functioning. Milk thistle prevents the depletion of glutathione, a substance that is crucial for the liver's role in detoxification. It also helps promote the regeneration of new liver cells. Alcohol depletes glutathione, but because of its antioxidant properties, milk thistle helps replenish glutathione. Glutathione is a cofactor for antioxidant enzymes and helps recycle other antioxidants, like vitamins C and E. *Dosage:* 400 mg per day.

Schisandra: Studies with animals suggest that schisandra may protect the liver from toxic damage, improve liver function, and stimulate cell regrowth in the liver. Schisandra seeds contain more than a dozen liver-protective compounds. It appears that schisandra lignans protect the liver by activating the enzymes in liver cells that produce glutathione, the liver's most important antioxidant. *Dosage:* 250 mg per day, either in tablet or liquid tincture form.

Before Bed, Try This:

- When you get home after a night of drinking, drink plenty of water before you go to bed. This will prevent the dehydration that accompanies most hangovers. A little Gatorade can also help you replace lost electrolytes, though it's not ideal because it contains high-fructose corn syrup, which is a cheaply processed, poor-quality sweetener.
- If you can remember, take 150 mg of milk thistle and 250 mg of schisandra. Before you go out, put them in the bathroom next to a big glass of water, so when you get home you won't forget.
- Also take 1,000 mg of N-acetyl cysteine and 500 mg of vitamin C.
- Take two 1,000-mg capsules of evening primrose oil, too.

The Morning After, Try This:

- Take 400 mg of magnesium as a rescue remedy.
- Take 1,000 mg of N-acetyl cysteine.
- Try 1,500–6,000 mg of MSM.
- For a sour stomach, take a heaping teaspoon of glutamine powder mixed into water.
- For headaches, you can try a natural aspirin remedy and take 800 mg of willow bark. Willow bark contains salicin, a substance used in aspirin. You can find it in a health-food store.
- Nux vomica in a homeopathic preparation will help relieve gas, bloating, and a sour stomach. Take the 6c potency in 4 drops or pellets every hour.
- Drink tomato juice. In addition to being a prevention remedy, tomato juice contains fructose, a type of sugar that helps your body metabolize alcohol more quickly. This is probably why the morning-after Bloody Mary seems to work.
- Eat crackers and honey. Honey has a high level of fructose and will be helpful in removing the remainder of the alcohol in your system. Fruit juice will do the same thing because of its high level of fructose.

SUGARPLUM FAIRIES

Japanese pickled plums, known as umeboshi plums, have remarkable medicinal qualities. Their powerful acidity has a paradoxical alkalinizing effect on the body, neutralizing fatigue, stimulating the digestion, and promoting the elimination of toxins. This is the Far Eastern equivalent to both aspirin and apple; not only is it a potent hangover remedy for mornings after but an umeboshi a day is regarded as the best preventive medicine available.

Umeboshi plums are available in jars at Oriental markets and natural-foods stores. They taste very salty. Japanese herbalists say the saltiness helps put the body back into balance by contracting the tissues that have overexpanded from too much alcohol. For a normal hangover, bite off about a quarter of a plum and keep it in your mouth until it dissolves. For a whopper hangover, herbalists recommend popping a whole plum in your mouth. Continue to suck on the pit for about an hour after the plum has dissolved.

- Refresh your sour palate with peppermint. The herb peppermint, taken either in tea form or by chewing the leaves, will relax the intestines. Peppermint is a carminative, which is a substance that removes accumulated gas from the stomach and intestines. Make a tea by pouring one cup of boiling water over 1–2 teaspoons of the dried herb; cover; steep for fifteen minutes; strain. Drink one or two cups as soon as you can.
- Last but not least, try having a soothing bath with sandalwood and lavender.

MIXING IT UP

Now that you know how to manage alcohol and its disruptive effects on the body, let's teach you to have fun with your drinks! Following are some classic concoctions and some new antioxidant-rich recipes that will give you a new place to rest your drink umbrella. Nothing makes a man stiffer than a gal who can make a stiff drink. Treat yourself to some basic yet classy accoutrements that you can keep on hand: a jigger, a shaker, an ice bucket, ice tongs, and a flask (for when you suspect there's going to be cheap booze at a party and you'll need to spike your drink with a treat from home. As you've learned, not all drinks are created equal; cheap liquors are far less distilled and therefore contain more impurities than their high-end counterparts, which can leave your head aching and put a damper on a fun night out). For you sassily sober babes, there's no need for you to feel left out here! Just grab yourself a mocktail and party on! Club soda with cranberry and lime, a virgin Bloody Mary, or a virgin cosmo served in a martini glass will look beautiful, taste delicious, and be consequence-free the morning after. Here's to drinking to your gorgeous self!

I've listed some standard drinks in the following pages so you'll have a few signature recipes for your repertoire. Feel free to pick up some bartending books or look online for fantastic recipes you might enjoy—the sky's the limit here! Both alcoholic and nonalcoholic drinks can create a theme and set the tone for parties. When you enter someone's home, nothing looks more inviting than a big pitcher of ice-cold drinks.

SHAKEN OR STIRRED?

Note to self: The martini is the perfect mixture of velvety vodka and olives, which are chock-full of essential fatty acids to help your liver metabolize it all. If you're making a martini or any drink you're going to be serving in a martini glass, it is imperative that you chill the glasses beforehand; this will keep the drink cold and remarkably smooth when it is served. Here are my tips for a no-fail martini: Fill the martini glasses with ice and water and set them in the freezer for two minutes while you're mixing the drinks. When you're ready to pour the mixed drink, pull the glasses out from the freezer and pour out the ice water. Your glasses will be chilled and ready to go! Also make sure you prep the bar area ahead of time: Slice up lemons and limes, fill the ice bucket, and keep toothpicks skewered with fat, juicy green cocktail olives in a highball glass so they can be plucked out and dunked right into your drink. *Voilà!*

Martini

1½ OUNCES VODKA

½ TEASPOON DRY VERMOUTH

3 COCKTAIL OLIVES

Pour the vodka into a shaker that is halfway filled with ice. Shake vigorously for 20 seconds; this will enable tiny ice crystals to form in the vodka. Set aside. Pour the dry vermouth into a martini glass. Swish the vermouth around the glass and shake the remnants out into the sink. Pour in the ice-cold vodka and add in the olives. If you like your martinis dirty, add in a splash of olive juice. If you prefer gin martinis, substitute gin for vodka and add in a pearl onion instead of the olives.

Bonus: Know how to make a martini and you will impress your guests.

Pomegranate Cosmos

¾ CUP VODKA

⅓ CUP TRIPLE SEC

⅓ CUP FRESH LIME JUICE

⅓ CUP POMEGRANATE JUICE

Fill a pitcher with ice. Add vodka, triple sec, fresh lime juice, and pomegranate juice. Stir until well combined and thoroughly chilled. Serve in martini glasses and garnish with a twist of lemon or lime.

Bonus: Pomegranate juice is chock-full of antioxidants, providing some protection for your cells while you drink.

Green Tea–Tini

1 OUNCE GREEN TEA, CHILLED

2 OUNCES GREY GOOSE CITRON VODKA

¼ OUNCE GRAND MARNIER

1 TEASPOON FRESH LIME JUICE

LIME SLICES FOR GARNISH

Pour the green tea, vodka, and Grand Marnier into a shaker that is halfway filled with ice. Shake vigorously for 20 seconds; this will enable tiny ice crystals to form in the vodka. Set aside. Pour the lime juice into a martini glass. Swish the lime juice around the glass and shake the remnants out into the sink. Pour the shaker ingredients into a martini glass and garnish with lime slices.

Bonus: Green tea is also loaded with polyphenols and antioxidants, improving the nutritional content of your alcoholic bevvie.

Gorgeous-tini

3 OUNCES LADY JANE PINK LEMONADE LIQUEUR

1 OUNCE STOLICHNAYA PEACH VODKA

LEMON PEEL TWIST, FOR GARNISH

Chill a martini glass in a refrigerator or freezer to give it that frosted look. Pour the Lady Jane Pink Lemonade and peach vodka into a shaker that is halfway filled with ice. Shake vigorously for 20 seconds; this will enable tiny ice crystals to form in the vodka. Pour into a martini glass and garnish with a lemon peel twist. For an extra sparkly touch, line the rim of the glass with pink sugar before you pour liquids in.

Bonus: While there may not be much nutritional value in this drink, Lady Jane is lower in sugar than most other liqueurs. Think of it as a celebration of your gorgeous self. You are so pretty in pink!

Mocktails

Pomegranate Mimosa

1 GLASS SPARKLING CIDER

½ OUNCE POMEGRANATE JUICE

LEMON PEEL FOR GARNISH

Pour sparkling cider into a champagne flute. Add the pomegranate juice. Use the lemon peel as a garnish you can drop right into the mimosa.

Bonus: This is a far more nutritious drink than soda, and is much prettier to look at!

BABY BELLINI
2 OUNCES PEACH NECTAR
1 OUNCE FRESH LEMON JUICE
CHILLED SPARKLING CIDER

Pour the peach nectar and the lemon juice into a chilled champagne flute. Stir well. Add cider to fill the remainder of the glass. Stir again gently.

Bonus: This also offers more benefits than soda and can be used as a virgin drink between alcoholic courses.

LAST CALL

Do some thinking before you go drinking. Don't drink on an empty stomach. Do drink water in between alcoholic cocktails. And remember to be a Gorgeous Girl—always the belle of the ball, never the belle of the bombed! Keep your act clean and you'll never have to explain yourself the next day or suffer with a bad hangover. The party life is much more of a party when you can get up off the couch the next day and get out to the places where your gorgeous face is needed: out shopping with the girls, or to the movies, a café, or the roller disco!

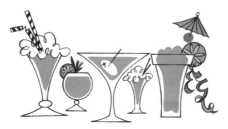

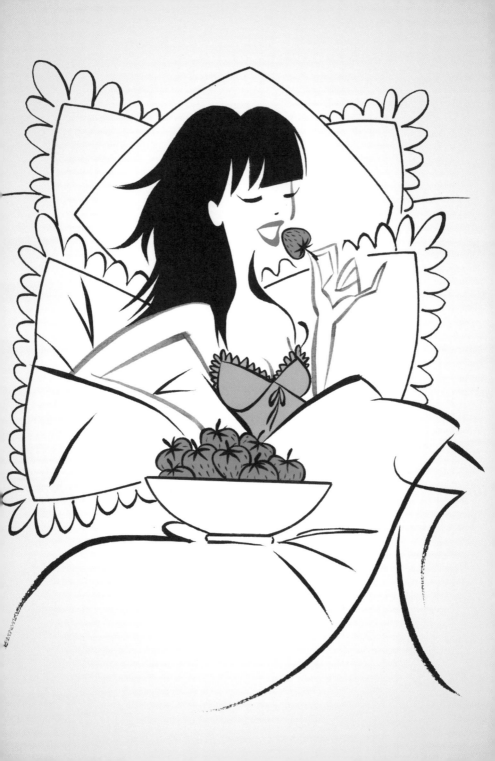

chapter 4

GORGEOUS
in Bed

I think I could fall madly in bed with you. –Unknown

Sure, good nutrition will give you gorgeous skin, a lean body, and great energy, but did you know that the right combinations of food and nutrients in supplement form can also make your sex life better? It's true. Just by eating a healthy diet, taking the right supplements, and taking care of your digestion you can increase your endurance and satisfaction and, most important, perform like the bucking bronco you know you are!

Believe me, I've heard it all. When people come into my practice, men and women alike, I often learn about their sex lives by default. I have heard tales of sexual woe that would give any cowgirl the blues—vaginal dryness, yeast infections, urinary tract infections, and sexually transmitted diseases can keep you locked up in the stables for quite some time and detract from a healthy libido. What many of my patients don't know, and what I'm here to tell you, is that sometimes the cure for what ails you could be right in your kitchen.

Most of us don't even realize that what we take in affects how we put out. In this chapter I'll outline what's best to eat before a hot date and what's best to eat for general sexual well-being. I'll provide information on which supplements can boost your libido and which foods work as aphrodisiacs. I'll also give you some pointers on how to eat to treat pesky conditions that can interfere with good lovin'.

Now, there are some conditions that healthful foods and supplements can't fix by themselves. If you have what you suspect is an STD, for instance, by all means consult your doctor. Or if you have a chronic condition that doesn't respond to my recommendations, seek out medical help.

Read on for some basics and some secrets to battling the pesky problems that can really bring a girl down, down there, so you can always feel gorgeous in bed.

FOOD FOREPLAY: INTER-COURSES

What to eat on a date? You're already a wee bit nervous. You might have butterflies in your stomach, so you may be tempted to go for a light salad or a ladylike bowl of pasta. But I'm here to tell you that a little meat (or some other form of protein, be it fish, chicken, or legumes) can go a long way. Of all the types of food, protein does the best job of keeping your blood sugar level. It gives you staying power, and will keep you cooking all night long. A big bowl of pasta could put you right to sleep, while a salad may not be enough to fill you up. So make sure that no matter what you order, it comes with some protein. Getting the right combination of protein, fat, and complex carbohydrates at each meal will stabilize your blood sugar for hours to come (no pun intended), because the combination of nutrients is much greater than the sum of its parts. For instance, when eaten together, steak, potatoes, and spinach break down much more slowly than just a plain old bowl of pasta would; without proteins or fats, white pasta is turned right into sugar and absorbed into the bloodstream instantly. So if you're hoping for a marathon session in bed, be sure you're properly fueled.

While you're going easy on the starches, make sure you go easy on high-fat foods, too—especially if you think you'll be getting lucky later on. Since fat takes the longest to digest, it will keep you feeling full for the greatest amount of time. I don't know about you, but I find it hard to feel romantic and sexy when I'm bloated, with a Buddha belly protruding out and slapping my honey to the other end of the bed! Men should bear in mind that eating too much fat at a meal lowers testosterone levels, decreases libido, and makes erection and ejaculation more difficult. So if you want to get lucky, persuade your man to eat light before sex. Which brings me to my next point: If you're going out for dinner together, don't stuff down a five-course meal with wine and dessert—at least not if you think you're going to have sex later on that night. It's best to finish eating dinner at least one hour before sex so you have properly digested. You can save your dessert course for bed.

It goes without saying that you should steer clear of gas-causing foods while on a date. Some of us have trouble digesting beans, tofu, milk, cheese, cream sauces, cabbage, broccoli, Brussels sprouts, prunes, apples, wheat products, fried foods, or carbonated drinks. Also be mindful of the combinations of foods you're eating. Believe it or not, fruit is easier to digest on an empty stomach than for dessert. Protein digests well with vegetables and fats, and carbohydrates digest well with vegetables and fats, but for some of our fartier friends, protein and carbohydrates don't always pair well together. If this is you, try having a steak with spinach for dinner, or go ethnic with lentils, rice, and veggies, but skip the chicken with rice and

WAXING PHILOSOPHICAL

While we're on the subject of eating out, let's pause for a moment and think about those of us who'll be *eating in*. If your man likes to explore your geography south of the border, keep your bush manicured. Picture yourself standing in sexy lingerie, about to be disrobed. Your lover kisses you, and gently begins to move to your nether regions. He pulls down the strings of your camisole. He kisses your neck. He loosens your panties and slowly slides them down. Wait, what does he see? Is it pleasing to the eye or a tad bit, er, unruly? Forgive me for being crass, but no man wants to go down on a woman who looks like a chimp in diapers! As a general rule, make sure your panties cover your thatch. If you're a natural gal who likes a fuller look or you're a career gal who's too busy to take care of her lady business, try some sassy boy-short panties. Whether you prefer a lush full patch, a neatly manicured landing strip, or a full-out Brazilian wax, keep it tidy and well-groomed and you'll keep him coming back.

veggies—your tender tummy just may not be up for the job of breaking down meat proteins and starches together.

Whatever you do, don't let these rules of thumb keep you from enjoying yourself and your food. There are tons of date-worthy foods that will keep your taste buds smiling. Eating sexy brings you pleasure, giving you a girly flush that emanates from within. Meow! When you're thinking about getting it on, think of sensual foods that turn you on. I'm Russian, so nothing gets me in the mood like blinis topped with caviar and crème fraîche, foie gras on toast points, and an extra-chilled martini. For others, it might be sucking down some oysters (rich in zinc and a natural aphrodisiac) with a big glass of wine, or rolling bread chunks in cheese fondue, or eating freshly washed grapes, one at a time, with a glass of Prosecco. Whatever it is that floats your boat, give these combinations of food a trial run before the date so you'll know how they sit in your system.

In terms of libations, drinking sexy will also give you pleasure, but don't overdo it; alcohol impairs sexual response by dulling the senses. Like caffeine, it appears to impair testosterone production, needed by both men and women for normal libido. Drinking a little less to feel a little more is a good trade-off, don't you think?

DIGESTIVE DO'S

Probably the last thing we want to think about in bed is digestion. It's just not very sexy. But poor digestion can seriously detract from the quality of your love life. I've said it before, and I'll say it again: I can't think of a better way to spruce up your love life than to take care of your digestive issues.

Because a healthy digestive tract is the foundation for good health, it has a domino effect on your organs and systems. The best way to keep your system running smoothly is with a high-fiber diet. The cleansing that comes from regular bowel movements (one to two times per day) prevents you from getting backed up and becoming a gassy lassie. Because let's face it: Nobody wants to let one rip while in the midst of an intimate moment. Talk about an embarrassment and a potential deal breaker! The same goes for those poor souls with irritable bowels; if the anticipation of a new date sets off stomach-churning bloating, gas, and diarrhea, then tuning up from the inside out

THE GARDEN OF EATING

If you like to entice a man with more than just the fruits of your loins, have I got some sweet treats for you! Bear in mind that none of these foods are low in calories or sugar...but, that's not exactly the point, now, is it? It's time for you to think outside the box (ahem) and introduce fun foods into your sex life:

- **Honey** will sweeten up your breasts and body and lead the bee right to your hive! Worried about stickiness? Trust me, it won't be on you long enough! For those who are carb-conscious, try **agave syrup**, which is derived from the nectar of the agave plant and looks and tastes like honey but is much lower in sugar.

- **Chocolate whipped cream** is the perfect topping for your sundae. Get the spray can, aim, and shoot!

- **Chocolate body paint:** Grab a paintbrush and run wild with your very own edible designs.

- For you Monica Lewinsky types, get up *in there* with some **candy canes**—the sticks are a refreshing after-dinner mint and you'll feel the cool breeze *everywhere!* If your man has Bill Clinton's charisma and charm but you're prone to yeast infections, try sucking on a candy cane and head south of the Beltway for some executive hanky-panky.

- Try using **cake frosting** while playing naked Twister. Loser must lick!

Note to self: Use your head when using food in bed. One poor soul was literally hard on her luck after her boyfriend decided she would taste much better dipped in butterscotch. So they melted butterscotch candies and poured the concoction on her mound, but before he was done eating, the butterscotch hardened up, and she wound up in the emergency room. And for you extra-adventuresome babes out there who battle yeast infections, please be mindful of putting sugary foods inside the vagina, which could worsen the situation. Proceed with caution and keep the treats for external use only!

should definitely be your first priority. And I'm going to tell you how. Trust me, you'll be doing all your potential suitors a big favor, and you'll save yourself a lot of grief down the road.

Smooth Moves

Although this isn't terribly sexy advice, I've got to say it anyway: It's crucial to get enough fiber in your diet on a daily basis. Adequate fiber will keep your system running smoothly and will offset the gas, bloating, and constipation that so many women suffer from. It will also decrease your risk of colon cancer and just keep you feeling better overall.

Fiber bulks up your stools and decreases the transit time of your bowel movements. If figuring out the amount of time it takes for food to pass through your system really turns you on, try this: Eat a cup of cooked beets. Keep an eye on your bowel movements until you find the one that is dark pink (yep, beets will do that to a girl), and you will be able to determine how long it took to get from point A to point B. Ideally this amount of time will be no more than twenty-four hours. But if you find that it takes more than twenty-four hours, get more fiber in your diet pronto.

Excellent high-fiber choices are freshly ground flaxseeds (three tablespoons provide 8 grams of fiber), dark green leafy vegetables, fresh fruits, beans and lentils, steel-cut oats, buckwheat, and barley. Ideally you should try to get 25 grams of fiber in your diet per day; the average American gets only 12 grams per day. Gasp! If you're constipated and addicted to flour-based products, remember this: Flour plus water makes paste! I can't tell you how many women have come into my practice moving their bowels only one to two times per week. But what I can tell you is that when I take them off processed foods and let them eat only whole foods, the situation changes—and for good. If you find that after cutting out the processed foods you still haven't seen the results you're hoping for, try taking 400 mg of magnesium chelate twice per day on an empty stomach to relax the bowels and let the poop out of the chute. Don't forget to drink at least six to eight glasses of water per day and get in some exercise, which also shakes things up and moves things along.

If you're at the other end of the spectrum and are crapping your brains out before a big date, try relaxing your nervous system and slowing things down by taking one tablespoon of L-glutamine powder mixed in water, along with a trace mineral formulation that contains calcium, magnesium, potassium, and iodine. Rescue Remedy is also a safe and gentle homeopathic that you can use a few times per day to help chill you out. You can even give it to your pets by putting it into their water when they need a chill pill.

PUTTING THE GAS MASK TO REST!

- Take acidophilus capsules or powder every day, especially if you are on oral contraceptive pills and or antibiotics. Make sure you take them with food. These will work to build "good bacteria" in your intestinal tract, which bulks up your bowel movements and enables them to pass through more quickly.

- Optimize your daily fiber intake. A high-fiber diet helps build "good bacteria" in your system, which in turn helps your body make digestive enzymes.

- Drink an adequate amount of water, herbal tea, or diluted juice to stay hydrated; at least 60 percent of constipation cases are due to dehydration. To figure out how much water you need, take your body weight in pounds and divide that number in half; that's how many ounces you'll need. For example, a 150-pound person would need 75 ounces of water, or about nine glasses per day. For every caffeinated drink you have, add another glass of water to your daily needs. During exercise, drink 4 to 8 ounces of water every twenty minutes.

- Eating bitter, dark green leafy vegetables, as well as beets, will help stimulate the digestive process and facilitate elimination.

LADIES, START YOUR ENGINES: SUPPLEMENTS

There are quite a few supplements you can take to enhance your sexual satisfaction. The natural solutions that follow can boost a low sex drive, produce essential hormones, direct blood to your sex organs, soften your skin, and bolster your immune system to help discourage STDs.

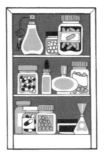

B Vitamins. These vitamins play best supporting actress in a woman's own personal love story. Your ability to react and respond to your leading man depends on how effectively your brain signals to your glands that it's time to initiate hormone production and the flow of blood to your sex organs. B vitamins are critical to the development of brain messengers for these signals. Vitamin B_6 is especially important because it prevents the over-production of prolactin, a libido saboteur. It also monitors your body's balance between estrogen and progesterone and reduces excess estrogen, which can cause severe PMS or perimenopausal mood swings in women. One hundred milligrams of B_6 per day will support hormonal balance and curtail those nasty mood swings. Incidentally, taking niacin, another B vitamin, thirty minutes before sexual activity can enhance your sexual flush by increasing blood flow to the skin and mucous membranes, intensifying your orgasm.

Bioflavonoids. Bioflavonoids play an important role in keeping blood vessels flexible and the uterus healthy, which is significant for women who have abnormal uterine bleeding. They also improve circulation to enhance whoopee potential. These vitamin-like substances are found in a wide variety of plants, especially grapes and pine tree bark.

Essential Fatty Acids. Essential fatty acids are the building blocks for the production of female sex hormones. They also help your body store more of the fat-soluble vitamins (like A, E, D, and K) that keep you sexually active. In addition, they provide moisture and softness to the skin, eyes, vagina, and bladder. Borage, primrose, flaxseed, and fish oils are available primarily in capsule form, though fresh flaxseeds and wild Alaskan salmon are also excellent sources of EFAs. See more about these incredible nutrients in the "Jiffy Lubing" section of this chapter.

Vitamin E. Vitamin E plays an important role in reproductive health. Found in foods such as olive oil, seeds and nuts, and organic butter, vitamin E can alleviate sexual problems like impotence and low sex drive. This powerful antioxidant protects your sex glands from the stress generated by free radicals. Free radicals are like loose cannons that can damage proteins, DNA, and the lipids inside the cells.

Zinc. The human sense of smell, which depends on the mineral zinc, is an oft-overlooked element in primal passion. Pheromones—in this case, the individual biological scent your body produces—can drive your lover wild. They're detected subconsciously but are a key element in sexual excitement. Unfortunately, in today's smell-phobic society the use of deodorants (and the contraceptive pill) seems to have interfered with our natural pheromone functions. So to keep your lover attracted to the real you, try using natural deodorants with a base of tea tree oil—they'll keep the bacteria at bay but let the true you shine through!

To tune in to your lover's pheromones, it's critical to make sure you're getting enough zinc-rich foods in your diet. Food-rich sources include oysters and other shellfish, turkey, mushrooms, and seeds like sesame, sunflower, poppy, and pumpkin. Also try sprouts, such as sunflower and alfalfa.

Added zinc bonus: Zinc-rich foods also increase sexual function in women. Zinc supports healthy adrenal activity, which combats the negative effects of stress. Healthy adrenals translate into more energy, and because you'll feel less burned out by physical activity, you'll benefit from increased sexual stamina. Zinc bolsters your immune function too, and may reduce your risk of contracting sexually transmitted diseases.

There you have it—the best supplements for your sexual health! Now, it should go without saying that supplements are no substitute for the vitamins and minerals found in good old-fashioned whole foods. Just because you take supplements doesn't mean you can skimp on the healthy foodstuffs. A gorgeous girl's diet is critical to her sexual prowess, her libido, and her sexual responsiveness. After all, who wants to be a cold fish in bed? A gland-boosting, hormone-balancing diet is critical to sexing it up. For you babes looking to add more sexual sparkle to your performance in the boudoir, do yourself a favor and include asparagus, cabbage, cauliflower, broccoli, tomatoes, squash, zucchini, carrots, peas, and yams in your diet—they'll give you enough energy-producing nutrients to keep you grinding all night long! Also get tropical with avocados, mangoes, papayas, citrus fruits, bananas, apples, pears, plums, peaches, and nectarines, which are chock-full of fiber, vitamins, and trace minerals to keep your blood sugar and your mood stable and happy. And make sure you have strawberries dipped in chocolate when duty calls! For a more comprehensive breakdown of dosages and protocols, see Chapter 5, "Vitamin G."

SALACIOUS SEX: APHRODISIACS

We've all heard that certain foods rev up your sex drive. While some of these foods have been scientifically proven to stimulate our systems, the others seem a bit funky. The following is a list of aphrodisiacs, some normal, and some…well, you be the judge! Figs, oysters, chocolate, asparagus, cheese, caviar, lobster, grapes, sardines, mushrooms, cinnamon, Spanish fly, and, last but not least, Rocky Mountain oysters (it doesn't matter what you call them—cooked right, testicles are a treat for some folks!) may increase your sexual prowess. You don't need to eat all these foods at once—lest you ruin a night of romance with some serious gas and indigestion!

HELL-ITOSIS: TIPS FOR IMPROVING YOUR BOUQUET

Has a funk cloud ever mysteriously descended upon you? Has anyone ever politely handed you mints so that you could clean up your abysmal breath? Have you ever discreetly lifted up your arm to sniff your pits, only to discover that your natural scent has been edged out by Eau de Roadkill? There isn't a person out there who hasn't succumbed to a little stinkiness now and then. It happens. But it's how you handle the stink—be it your armpits, breath, or vagina—that makes all the difference.

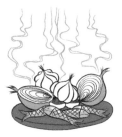

BREATH

Halitosis is often caused by a buildup of bacteria within the mouth—from food debris, plaque, or gum disease—or in a coating on the back of the tongue. Good oral hygiene will usually solve the problem. Keep up with regular brushing of your teeth and tongue, flossing, and antiseptic mouthwashes. Eating clean, fresh foods and cutting back on dairy will also fight bad breath, since dairy often produces extra mucus in the intestinal tract. Try to be aware of odiferous foods: If they smell to you, then they will smell to others! Garlic, onions, and sardines are just a few likely offenders. A good rule of thumb is to do as your date does. If he requests no onions on his burger, by all means, follow suit.

But let's say you're a risk taker on a date. The menu comes, and what jumps right out at you but the linguine with clam sauce and extra garlic. Loaded with ammunition, you don't stop there; you order the garlic bread and a big glass of wine to polish it all off. You enjoy every bite, licking your chops, your napkin greasy with butter stains and stray bits of chopped garlic. At the end of the meal, your date is aroused by your hearty appetite, and leans across the table to plant a smooch on your lubricated lips. But before he gets there, a virtual punch in the face of unadulterated zest hits him, making him recoil in horror! Don't fear, my dear: Relief is just a parsley sprig away. Find the garnish on your plate and chew it down. Parsley is particularly good for cleansing the palate, but if you feel that it's too conspicuous, order some sorbet after dinner to refresh your kisser. And at the end of the meal, regardless of what you eat, grab some mints pronto! Don't mess around here and leave things to fate; stay prepared so you can pucker up on quick notice. The flip side to carrying mints is that if your date has a stinky flytrap, you can freshen up together.

Armpits

For stinky pits, try a natural deodorant containing tea tree oil or baking soda. Tea tree oil has antibacterial properties, and baking soda also mops up bad odors. On the days you wake up in time to shower and apply deodorant before you get to work, these natural remedies will do the trick of keeping your stench at bay. But what happens when you've been out until the wee hours of the morning and barely have time to change for work, let alone shower? Or when you leave work in a fluster, trying to squeeze in a workout before heading out for a night on the town, knowing that having enough time to shower afterward will be an impossible feat? In either case, you must incorporate what some call the "whore's bath" into your regime: Grab a washcloth lathered up with some gentle cleanser and give your armpits and vaginal region a quick once-over. That will clean the barest of essentials while offsetting anything offensive. And if your hair is slightly greasy or sweaty, polish off your look with a mixture of conditioner and gel and slick it back into a ponytail gathered at the nape of your neck. Gorgeous you!

Vagina

If you are self-conscious about the way your vagina smells, take some simple steps to improve the situation. First and foremost: Wear cotton undies, don't sit around in wet clothes, and skip the underwear at night. Let yourself air out and your vagina will repay you in kind. In the shower, use a very gentle cleanser and don't oversoap yourself, which can be very irritating to the delicate tissue in the area and can cause changes in pH balance that can worsen yeast infections.

If you're feeling not-so-fresh, you may be tempted to douche. I don't recommend it. All healthy vaginas contain some bacteria and other organisms, called the vaginal flora. The normal acidity of the vagina keeps the amount of bacteria down. Douching can change this delicate balance by decreasing the acidity of the vagina—ultimately making a woman more prone to vaginal infections. Plus, douching can introduce new bacteria up into the uterus, fallopian tubes, and ovaries.

Last but not least, know your scent. If there's something amiss down there and lately there haven't been any takers for your bouquet, hustle on over to the gyno's office and get things checked out. A change in odor that is reminiscent of last night's fish dinner could be caused by bacterial vaginosis (read on in this chapter for more information).

JIFFY LUBING: DO YOU NEED AN OIL CHANGE?

Our personal lubrication fluctuates throughout our cycles. But for some, vaginal dryness is a persistent problem. It's usually caused by hormonal shifts that thin the vaginal walls and decrease the quantity of normal lubrication. You may find that this is something you've dealt with all your life, and by now you've invested stock in Astroglide and K-Y Jelly. But did you know that you can dramatically turn things around by getting the right fats in your diet? The 1980s trained us to avoid fats, which did a huge disservice to Americans at the public health level. We need fats to balance out our blood sugar and our mood and to help us stay lean and mean. Healthy fats such as olive oil, nuts and seeds, and avocados also contain natural lubricants that are crucial for the formation of hormones. Cholesterol is actually a precursor for hormones; if a woman does not have enough body fat, she may suffer from vaginal dryness and have painful sex as a result. Also, fats and cholesterol actually regulate your hormones from a very early age by making estrogen, progesterone, and testosterone. Without these essential fats, hormonal imbalances can occur, and the body won't develop properly.

We truly are what we eat. The fats that we put into our bodies have powerful regulatory mechanisms that control menstrual regularity, inflammation (a response of body tissues to injury or irritation), and how we store our own body fat and metabolize our blood sugar. Buyers beware here: Hydrogenated oils, found in margarine, fried foods, and commercially baked goods, can wreak havoc on your health and begin the inflammatory cascade. Those fats will not only raise your cholesterol but will actually decrease your body's ability to metabolize sugars properly and can cause you to gain weight! Hydrogenated oils also block your body's normal healthy breakdown of fats and can cause inflammation within your body, such as menstrual cramps, headaches, breast tumors, and polycystic ovarian disease. So please do a reality check on your diet and look at what kinds of fats you are putting into your body. If you eat any processed foods whatsoever, try to eliminate them or find a healthier version. If you're suffering from any of the complaints mentioned previously, you need an oil change!

So what to do about dry sex? Here are some simple remedies: First and foremost, eating healthful fats is essential. If you have a lifetime of eating poor-quality fats and you suddenly clean out the riffraff, give your body *at least one year* to displace all the unhealthy fats with the healthy ones at the cellular level. If it seems shocking that it could take this long to produce results, don't feel discouraged. Remember that fat cells release toxins very slowly, so just give your body time to change at the cellular level. Even small changes in your diet will yield big results.

- Take at least 1–2 tablespoons of flaxseed oil every day. Flaxseed oil is rich in omega-3 fats, which are the same fats found in fish oils. Omega-3 fats are natural lubricants for your body, as they moisturize you from the inside out. Why is it that we spend so much money on unctions, lotions, and potions to correct dry skin, without even wondering why our skin is dry? The same thing goes for internal lubrication. The first and foremost cause of vaginal dryness is a deficiency in essential fatty acids. If your vagina is the lock, flaxseed oil is the key!

- You can also alternate flaxseed oil with cod liver oil to boost your immune system. Don't try just any old nasty-tasting fish oil, mind you; look for lemon-flavored oil, which doesn't have a hint of fishiness once it's refrigerated. Cod liver oil is rich in omega-3 fats, as well as vitamins A and D. Omega-3 fats decrease blood pressure, lower cholesterol, help prevent blood clots, improve menstrual regularity, ease menstrual cramps and headaches, and promote weight loss. Omega-3 fats are metabolically active and are quickly used for energy, rather than being stored as fat.

- For symptomatic relief, insert a wheat-germ-oil gelcap into the vagina; this remedy is safe and gentle enough to use even if you're prone to yeast infections. Wheat-germ oil is rich in vitamin E and will help re-create natural lubrication. You can insert it up to one hour before intercourse. As it warms up to your body temperature, the gelcap will dissolve and leave behind a silky residue. And it doesn't just feel good—it tastes good too! You can take wheat-germ oil orally for results as well.

SEXERCISE: TRAINING FOR THE BIG EVENT

What are some other things you can do to enhance your love life? For one thing, get your rear in gear and work it out! Not surprisingly, people who work out regularly have better sex lives. Intercourse and exercise are both athletic events, so this makes perfect sense. It is highly debated among athletes whether or not it's better to have sex before or after exercise. If you're planning on a sexual activity right *after* an endurance event, a serious power nap might be in order first! But hey, if you're an acrobat in the boudoir and really like athletic post-exercise sex, then let your partner know it's your turn to be on the bottom so you can rest your tired dogs while doing it doggy-style!

No chapter about sex would be complete without a discussion on Kegel exercises, which do both men and women's bodies good! (For you Jewesses out there, these are not to be confused with Kugel exercises.) A Kegel is a pelvic-floor exercise named after Dr. Arnold Kegel, who discovered it. (I would have liked him as my lab partner!) Both men and women have a PC (pubococcygeus) muscle, which is responsible for the tone and function of the pelvic floor. But trust me, that's not all it's used for. Keeping this muscle in tip-top shape will strengthen erections and improve orgasms. See page 92 for tips on Kegel excercises.

To locate the muscle, the next time you go to the bathroom, try to stop the flow of urine midway. Can you? If not, then you need to start exercising as soon as possible to maintain your inner fitness. Just as working out your biceps will give you better definition and more strength, working the PC muscle can help you strengthen and better define your orgasms. But as is the case with everything, due diligence is required. Remember that the stronger your PC muscle is, the more enjoyable sex will ultimately be!

Keep in mind that you can do these exercises just about anywhere and at any time, so there is absolutely no excuse to neglect them. No one will know that you're squeezing—unless, of course, you keep smiling like an idiot while doing them. Let's begin exercising, shall we?

THE PILL CAN BE A REAL PILL

For many women, the pill is a practical, convenient, and reliable source of contraception. By overriding the body's natural ovulation cycles, the pill

PUNANI POWER

Beginner: Baby Steps

1. Quickly clench your PC muscle and hold for 10 seconds; rest for 10 seconds and then repeat. Perform 3 sets and then take a 30-second break.

2. Clench your PC muscle and hold for 5 seconds; rest for 5 seconds. Repeat 10 times.

3. Clench your PC muscle and hold for 30 seconds; rest for 30 seconds. Repeat 3 times.

4. Repeat the first step and you're done for the day.

Intermediate: Glamma-Puss

1. Clench your PC muscle and hold for 5 seconds; release. Repeat 10 times.

2. Squeeze and release the muscle 10 times quickly. Do 3 sets.

3. Clench and release your PC muscle, alternating long counts of 10 with short counts of 10. Repeat 3 times.

4. Squeeze your PC muscle and hold it for as long as you can. Try to work your way up to 120 seconds. (Relax, that's only two minutes.)

Advanced: Ride 'Em, Cowgirl!

1. Fully squeeze and release your PC muscle over and over again. Begin with one set of 30; slowly work your way up to over 100.

2. Squeeze your PC muscle as tightly as you possibly can. (Make sure it's only your PC muscle that you're clenching, not your PC and abdominals.) Hold it for 20 seconds, then rest for 30 seconds. Repeat 5 times.

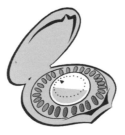

makes the chance of becoming pregnant extremely low. However, the pill is not without its risks and downsides; anytime you mess with Mother Nature she can mess right back with you. Fortunately, there are a few preventive measures that can help you combat her wrath.

Research has shown that regular usage of the pill can deplete the body's stores of vitamin B_6, which is critical for healthy nerve function, water balance, and the production of serotonin and dopamine. Serotonin and dopamine are powerful neurotransmitters that help keep us happy and calm. In fact, without them we can become quite depressed, crave sugars, and may need antidepressants. So buyer beware: If you are on the pill, supplement with at least 50 mg of B_6 per day.

You should also be aware that recent studies show that women who take a birth control pill might increase their risk of cervical and breast cancer. While oral contraceptives protect against some types of cancer, they can trigger others. Liver cancer has previously been indicated as a risk for women who take the pill. If you choose the pill as your method of birth control, discuss the risks and benefits with your doctor.

The pill can also exacerbate systemic yeast overgrowth. I've counseled countless women with very stubborn yeast and sinus infections who have a very long history of oral contraceptive use. So if you're gonna pop the hormones every day, you'll need to supplement with probiotics, which are the beneficial bacteria found in our intestinal tracts. Taking probiotics regularly promotes healthy gut function and fights yeast overgrowth by sustaining the good bacteria in your system. In turn, this helps ensure that yeast levels do not get out of control. Everyone who is on the pill needs to take probiotics every day; powder or pills are fine, just aim for a count of eight billion organisms per day. Eating yogurt and kefir will also be helpful.

One more word to the wise, and I have to say it: Use condoms regardless of whether or not you are taking the pill! There are an awful lot of STDs out there, and slipping a raincoat on your man's johnson takes all of about five seconds (trust me, I've mastered it), so no excuses. A lifetime of managing a potentially fatal and socially stigmatized disease just ain't worth it. It also deserves mention here that a latex barrier on your man's manhood will help prevent the two of you from giving each other the gift that keeps on giving. That's right, ladies—a condom really is the way to go when you want to avoid passing yeast back and forth between the two of you. And after sex, don't forget to urinate, wipe front to back, and clean yourself off with a warm washcloth. A gentle cleanser like Cetaphil can get rid of stubborn bacteria or irritating spermicide without disrupting the delicate pH of your dainty areas.

THE YEAST BEAST

Do you know any women who have *not* had at least one yeast infection? Neither do I! Unfortunately, at one time or another, every girl goes through a week of pain, itching, burning, messy creams, and circumstantially imposed abstinence due to a yeast infection. If you have suffered from a yeast infection only once or twice in your life, consider yourself lucky; I get scores of women coming into my practice who have them every month, some for weeks at a time! I can't think of anything less fun or more frustrating. Be sure to tell your beau about this part of the chapter, as yeast infections can be passed back and forth between couples! In the most serious cases I've seen in practice, I have had to treat both partners of a team to cover all the bases and facilitate healing.

What causes yeast infections? There are a host of factors that can alter your body's natural state of well-being. Nowadays, the bacteria inside the intestinal tract, or gut, are considered to be their own separate organ. These bacteria weigh about three to four pounds, amounting to billions of bacteria that keep the immune system functioning normally. Every day we naturally shed and turn over some of those bacteria through our bowel movements, and more colonize in their place. Both men and women have "good" bacteria and "bad" bacteria that maintain an intricate balance within the gut. Certain lifestyle factors can disrupt this delicate balance, and should be addressed accordingly.

BACTERIAL VAGINOSIS:
THERE'S SOMETHING FISHY GOING ON

Bacterial vaginosis is an infection caused by an overgrowth of the bacteria that are normally present in the vagina. Although it is more common in women who are sexually active, it also occurs in women who are not sexually active (self-pleasuring doesn't count here!). Like yeast infections, the symptoms often include a discharge, which can have a fishy smell. Vaginosis can be treated with medication, either topical or oral, prescribed by your doctor. I also recommend that you take a heaping teaspoon of acidophilus powder to recalibrate your vaginal habitat and for long-term prevention.

ALCOHOL: LIQUID BREAD

All alcohols are fermented and, therefore, contain yeast. So putting yeasted drinks in your body if you're already prone to yeast infections just isn't the best idea. Beer is by far the worst offender; you're basically drinking liquid bread. Wine falls second in line, leaving hard alcohols as your best bet. I'm a big fan of vodka, which is pretty pure and clean. Mixed with a splash of lime juice, on the rocks, or thrown in with club soda and lime wedges does me justice. But don't go overboard. One or two glasses will help you get your groove on and keep your buzz without the hideous hangover the next day.

ANTIBIOTICS: THE QUICK FIX?

We all know that antibiotics are a fast solution to nagging infections, but in the long run they can cause more harm than good. For those of you who pop them like candy, *faites-attention* here—the Latin root of the word *antibiotic* literally means "against life"! Picture this scenario: You are an unfortunate victim of chronic sinus infections, which are simply yeast infections that have moved farther north. Your head aches, your sinuses are clogged, and your nose is raw and runny. You go to the doctor, who can prescribe you an antibiotic to relieve your symptoms. After four days and nights of not sleeping, you concede and break out the pills; after all, life must go on, right? One Z-pack later and you're out on the town, partying it up with the gals again, only to come down with yet another infection the following week. Does this remind you of anyone you know? If so, you need to rethink your relationship with your body and why you got the darned infection in the first place. Now, believe me, there is a time and a place for antibiotics, so I don't want to knock them altogether. But if you're using them once a year or more, that should be a wake-up call that your immune system needs a jump start.

Often the root cause of yeast infections is the overuse of antibiotics (either as an adult or as a child), birth control pills, a high-sugar diet, stress, or poor hygiene practices. So the best way to treat the infections is through lifestyle management, because once you have a yeast infection you will always be prone to them. If you are prone to sinus infections, it would behoove you to invest in a Neti Pot (or as I fondly call it, the Snot Pot). Neti Pots resemble Hobbit-sized teapots that can be filled with a saline solution, which is then poured through your nasal cavities. Sounds unglamorous, I know, but regular nasal lavage will treat the symptoms of a sinus infection and provide much-needed relief without your having to resort to antibiotics and their resultant yeast infections. As for vaginal yeast infections, a whole-foods diet rich in unrefined foods and fiber is the way to go. Garlic, yogurt, and flaxseeds are all functional foods that can help create a healthy gut environment, which makes it far more difficult for yeast to thrive.

THERE'S A FUNGUS AMONG US

- If you are on the pill, make sure you take 50 mg of vitamin B_6 per day and probiotics in powder or capsule form; aim for a count of eight billion organisms per day.

- Cook with garlic and coconut oil, which are natural antifungals that fight yeast.

- Use condoms and practice good hygiene after sex.

- Look out for the yeastier alcoholic drinks, like wine and beer; stick to hard alcohols with a splash of club soda and lime.

STDs AND UTIs: RELIEF ASAP!

Herpes, Dysplasia, and Warts—Oh My!

Herpes, cervical dysplasia, and genital warts (caused by the human papilloma virus, or HPV) run rampant within most of our coochies, and most of us don't even know it! According to an article published in 1997 in the *American Journal of Medicine,* about 74 percent of Americans—nearly three out of four—have been infected with genital HPV at some point in their lives. HPV is the cause of abnormal Pap smears and genital warts. While you can be a lifelong carrier, you may not show any other signs or symptoms.

It's true that most often genital HPV produces no symptoms or illness, and so a person who has been infected may never know about it. Experts estimate that at any given time, only about 1 percent of all sexually active Americans have visible genital warts. Far more women have abnormal Pap smears related to HPV infection, but in many cases health-care providers do not explain the link between HPV and cervical infection, perpetuating the misunderstanding.

About 50 to 80 percent of American adults have oral herpes, which produces what are commonly called cold sores or fever blisters. About one in four adults in the United States has genital herpes. However, most people don't know they are infected because their symptoms are too mild to notice or are mistaken for another condition.

YOU BOOZE, YOU LOSE (YOUR COMMON SENSE, THAT IS)

As tempting as it may be to go out on a date and get smashed with a little Nerve Clicquot, try to keep the booze to a minimum. Alcohol may loosen you up, but it can also make you forget about things like having safe sex and performing well. Most of my patients have or have been exposed to at least one STD in their years in the dating world. So while booze may take the edge off a potentially awkward first sexual encounter, try to at least have one sober conversation ahead of time to avoid any unwanted gifts.

The most serious risk to our bodies from herpes and genital warts is a higher risk of cervical cancer. But with the proper treatment, most of us can live long and happy lives without any serious ramifications. No matter what the severity is, though, don't mess around with these conditions. Be diligent about getting regular gynecological checkups and Pap smears one or two times per year, as both a preventative measure and to monitor any changes in cervical cells. If you suffer from one of these STDs, fear not, my sweet girl—there are things you can do to ease the pain.

Herpes: Boosting the immune system with nutrients that have antiviral properties can help your body fight the good fight: olive leaf extract, vitamin C, St. John's wort, and echinacea have a powerful effect on the body that will help keep herpes symptoms at bay. L-lysine has also been shown to be effective against herpes by improving the balance of nutrients necessary to reduce viral growth of the herpes virus.

Avoid soy, nuts and seeds, sugar, and alcohol during active herpes outbreaks. Sugar and alcohol will wear down your immune system, and soy, nuts, and seeds are very high in arginine, an amino acid that can counteract the effects of lysine. Lysine is an amino acid that suppresses the signs and symptoms of herpes.

Dysplasia and Genital Warts: For dysplasia and genital warts, use the HPV Soothers below from your first diagnosis until your next Pap smear, which should be done six months later. The nutrients listed below should help normalize your cervical cells.

HPV SOOTHERS

Beta Carotene: 50,000 IU per day for six months—make sure it's from a food-based formula (see Chapter 5, "Vitamin G," for more information on food-based complexes).

Folic Acid: 20 mg per day for six months.

Echinacea: 1 teaspoon of liquid extract (from *Echinacea purpurea* root 1:2 extract) diluted in a shot of water or juice; take once a day for six months.

Last but not least, don't forget to keep yourself updated on the most cutting-edge facts and figures about STDs by logging on to the American Social Health Association's Web site, www.ashastd.org. If you already have herpes or an STD, try visiting the online dating Web site www.mpwh.org. If you can't beat 'em, join 'em!

UTIs (Urinary Tract Infections)

A UTI is an infection anywhere in the urinary tract. Your urinary tract includes the kidneys, ureters, bladder, and urethra. The urinary tract is the body's filtering system for removal of liquid wastes. Women are especially susceptible to bacteria, which may invade the urinary tract and multiply, resulting in infection. During sex, bacteria can enter the urethra and travel to the bladder and kidneys. In most cases, your body removes the bacteria, and you have no symptoms. Some women seem to be more prone to infection than others; it can become a frustrating battle.

UTIs can be pesky and painful reminders that you've just indulged in a wild sexfest. Honeymooners out there, beware! To keep bacteria away from your urethra, make sure you pee after having sex and wipe yourself front to back. The same goes for bowel movements—clean yourself up well, because the bacteria that cause UTIs live in your intestines, so pooping with poor hygiene can lead to a UTI. Fortunately, there are natural remedies (see page 100) that will treat your UTI and let you avoid using antibiotics.

HERPES SOOTHERS

Olive Leaf Extract: 500 mg (Olea europaea leaf standardized to 6% [30 mg] oleuropein); take 4 capsules every 3 hours, up to 16 a day.

L-lysine: 500 mg; take 6 capsules twice per day.

Vitamin C: 1,000 mg three times per day.

St. John's wort (from *Hypericum perforatum* flowering herb 2.5 g): take 1 teaspoon diluted in a shot of water or juice.

Echinacea (from *Echinacea purpurea* root 1:2 extract): 1 teaspoon diluted in a shot of water or juice.

Calcium lactate: 250 mg twice per day

UTIs AND CYSTITIS SOOTHERS

D-Mannose Powder: Take 1 teaspoon in water every 3 hours for the first 2 days. On day 3, take 1 teaspoon 3 times per day. On day 4, take just 1 teaspoon. The maintenance dose is 1 teaspoon per day. Drink a *lot* of water. D-mannose prevents *E. coli* bacteria from sticking to the bladder walls.

Cranberry Concentrate (cranberry fruit juice concentrate in a 25:1 formulation): Take 2 tablets 3 or 4 times per day for acute infections and 1 tablet 3 or 4 times per day for chronic infections. Take 1 tablet 3 times per day as a maintenance dose.

Uva-ursi Leaf (500 mg in a 4:1 extract): Take 2 tablets 3 or 4 times per day for acute infections and 1 tablet 3 or 4 times per day for chronic infections. Take 1 tablet 3 times per day as a maintenance dose.

PUT THE SWING IN HIS DING

So, what about the men in our lives? There are plenty of supplements and strategies to keep their reproductive regions healthy and fit. Recent research shows that omega-3 fats are the must-have of good nutrition not only for women but for our menfolk, too. Freshly ground flaxseeds are an especially good source of omega-3 fats for men. Flaxseeds are rich in lignans, which are the insoluble fibers that help protect against both breast and prostate cancer. Three tablespoons of flax meal provides 8 grams of fiber, and it's easy to sprinkle on yogurt, protein smoothies, oatmeal, and salads. (Some of my patients even sprinkle it on their ice cream!) At roughly a dollar per pound, flax meal is cost-effective. And don't forget about a wonderful source of omega-3 fats: fish and fish-oil supplements, which I'll talk more about in Chapter 5, "Vitamin G." If he eats wild cold-water fatty fish, such as wild Alaskan salmon or sardines, three to five times per week, it will help promote circulation throughout his body—especially to all the crucial areas where every ounce of blood counts!

If you need to address your man's low sex drive, think zinc! Ever hear that oysters are an aphrodisiac? Well, no surprise there: Oysters are rich in

NUTRIENTS AND TIPS TO
INCREASE YOUR MAN'S MOJO

For a low sex drive, it would be prudent for your beau to go to a doctor and get his testosterone and DHEA levels checked to rule out any organic causes of loss of randiness. The root cause of a low sex drive may be low hormonal levels brought on by stress or environmental toxins. Remember to chill out; stress inhibits the production of serotonin, which affects sperm counts and ejaculations.

- **Zinc:** Take 25–50 mg per day. Zinc needs to be balanced with copper, a vital mineral for heart health, so for long-term zinc supplementation take 3 mg of copper per day.

- **CoQ10:** Take 100 mg per day. CoQ10 helps improve fertility and sperm production. The best side effect of CoQ10 is increased energy and endurance—and who couldn't use more of that?

- **Tribulus:** Take 1 tsp. of liquid extract per day. Tribulus is a wonderful herb that improves sex drive, endurance, and fertility for both men and women. You should buy this through a nutritionist or nutritionally oriented physician who carries reputable brands in his or her practice.

For chronic problems with impotence and erectile dysfunction, visit the doctor to get checked out for diabetes and/or heart disease. Poor blood flow to the reproductive organs could be the result of clogged plumbing.

zinc, which helps make testosterone and subsequently puts a little schwing in his schlong. About 25 mg per day is sufficient for a maintenance dose, but if your man eats a diet high in sugar and/or refined carbs (pasta, white rice, milk, cookies, white bread, and white potatoes), his zinc levels will probably be low, so you should suggest 50 mg per day for about three months to get him up to speed. Zinc is one of the many trace minerals in our bodies that help regulate blood sugar balance, so eating an excess amount of carbohydrates and starches naturally depletes the body's reserves.

GETTING A HEART-ON

Now that you're starting to realize the effect nutrition can have on your love life, here's another tip: Healthy hearts make for healthy penises. In fact, the johnson can be a powerful diagnostic tool to the inner workings of the body. The penis contains thousands of microvessels that engorge with blood when duty calls. As we age, many factors can influence a man's performance and erectile ability, including hormonal fluctuations, stress, and dietary habits. It's no big surprise that diet plays an incredibly important role here. If you find that your partner isn't exerting his usual amount of stamina or, worse yet, can't even get it up, head straight to the doctor to rule out some potentially serious medical problems, such as heart disease and diabetes.

You may be thinking, What does my man's willy have to do with heart disease and diabetes? Like a newly dating couple, the two often go hand in hand. People with poorly controlled diabetes have sugar molecules pumping through their vessels for hours after they eat a meal. Over time, the sugar begins to cause permanent damage to the blood vessels, impairing the circulation and the body's ability to heal itself in those areas. The hands, feet, eyes, kidneys, heart, brain, and sex organs all suffer the brunt of the disease, as their blood supply is fed by the tiniest and most fragile capillaries and blood vessels. So if your man's peter is petering out, it could be a window into a more serious issue that should definitely get checked out. The same rule goes for heart disease and erectile function; if the main coronary arteries are clogged, it will decrease blood flow to the rest of the body. That's a heart attack waiting to happen and a recipe for poor sex life, to boot.

One last noteworthy tip: When it comes to heart disease and risk of diabetes, check out your man's gut-butt ratio; if his gut sticks out more than his butt does, he's at high risk for health problems down the road. A big gut coupled with no-ass-at-all is the body's way of saying it can't handle the breakdown of sugars, which can turn into diabetes if left untreated, and ultimately put him at risk for a heart attack.

YOU'VE MADE YOUR BED; NOW YOU GET TO LIE IN IT

So there you have it: everything you ever wanted to know about what to eat to amp up your sex life. Armed with all this good info, you're sure to really enjoy yourself and your man. Although you may hit a few bumps in the road, it's pretty standard and just the small price wild women pay for all the fun to be had! Just keep your head on straight and your vagina healthy, and you'll always be gorgeous in bed.

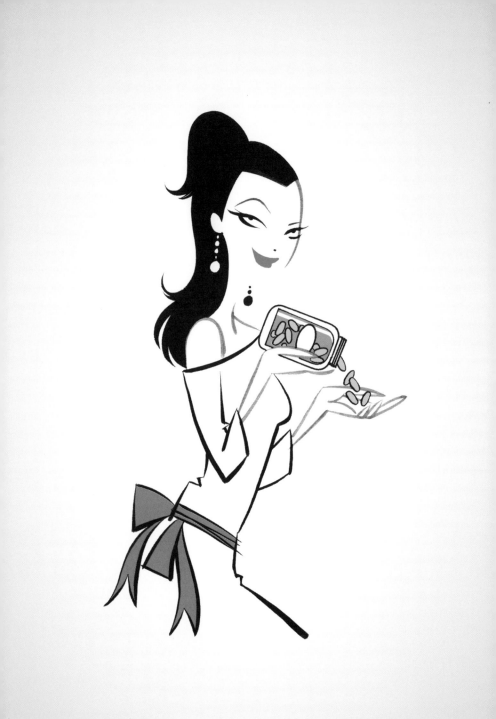

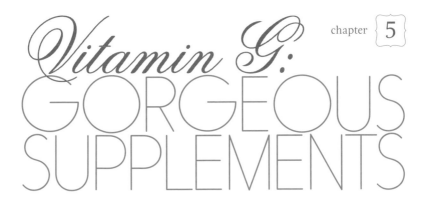

Vitamin G: GORGEOUS SUPPLEMENTS

chapter 5

In nature, nothing is perfect and everything is perfect. —Alice Walker

Eating a healthy diet without taking supplements is like wearing a ball gown without the right accessories; without the right look of one, the other is a disaster. This chapter explains why you should take supplements, which ones to take, and which types are absorbed best. To make things easy-breezy, I've organized all the information by ailment. Say you're feeling a little blue: Just flip to the entry for depression to find out how to put some pep back in your step. Got a pesky bladder infection? Turn to the UTI entry for info on how to take the sting out of your thing. I've included the most common complaints I hear about in my practice. Colds and flus, PMS, acne, constipation—it's all here. It's a terrible shame to waste precious moments feeling unwell. Follow my advice and you'll be back on your feet again in no time flat! If you're not familiar with some of the supplements listed, don't worry your pretty head; I've included a glossary at the end of the book so you can get the 411 on what you're taking.

A word to the wise here: Never take any medications, especially MAO inhibitors, with grapefruit juice. Doing so will increase the rate at which the medication is excreted from your system, decreasing the time it stays in your system and, ultimately, its efficacy. And *none* of the information listed in this chapter is meant to be a substitute for expert medical advice.

TO VITAMIN B OR NOT TO VITAMIN B

Are supplements truly necessary? Yes! I truly believe that in today's day and age, supplements are absolutely necessary. Think about the pace at which we live our lives. We put our bodies under a good deal more stress than our ancestors ever did. Working long hours, staring at computer screens, eating processed foods, drinking cosmos, *and* leading a glamorous nightlife take their toll, increasing the nutritional demands on our bodies and taxing our systems.

On top of all this, today's soils are often overfarmed, leaving them deficient in trace minerals. As a result, our fruits, vegetables, and grains have much less nutritional value than foodstuffs from a few generations ago. It's true that organic foods have significantly higher nutrient levels than commercially farmed foods, but keep in mind that even organic foods lose their nutrients if not eaten while fresh. What happens if the organic vegetables come from the West Coast and you live on the East Coast? Most likely they were harvested five days before they reached the grocery store, and it could be another three before you purchase them, which ensures vitamin losses before you've even cooked the darn things, and, well, you get my point.

Now, before you get completely depressed and throw in the towel, remember that there is still a lot you can do for yourself with a combination of eating right, relaxing, and taking supplements. Take me, for instance. I don't insist that everything I eat be organic; organic foods are not always available, and I would probably have to take out a second mortgage on my apartment to afford it all! The good news is that no matter whether your fruits and veggies are organic or not, they're still fruits and veggies and still a heck of a lot healthier than a bag of chips or 32-ounce soda. Every little healthy thing you do does indeed help, and you don't have to do it perfectly, either. By no means is my diet perfect every single day, and that is why I take supplements.

A–B–C EASY AS 1-2-3

So what kinds of vitamins should you take? I'm going to get to that. But first, a word on the different types: food-based and synthetic. Food-based supplements are advantageous because they contain the whole-food complex and as a result can be effectively assimilated into the body at a lower dose and with a higher efficacy. They contain enzymes, coenzymes, antioxidants, and trace elements that make them biologically available and improve absorption by the body. You can buy them from health-care practitioners and at specialty supplement stores. Synthetic supplements are the most common types of supplements available. They are manufactured in a laboratory and have druglike effects on the body, because they are acting in isolation and do not contain the vitamin cofactors found in their whole-food counterparts. However, synthetic supplements, which are not readily available in nature, have beneficial therapeutic uses in treating health problems. When I want to work more aggressively at treating a chronic health condition, I will incorporate synthetic supplements, such as alpha lipoic acid, into my treatment protocol.

Please bear in mind that the protocols listed below are not intended to diagnose a condition, treat it, or replace the recommendations of your doctor; nor are they meant to provide medical advice. They are simply guidelines for natural remedies to treat what ails you. So please run these by your nutritionally oriented physician before trying them. You do not have to take all of the supplements if you do not want to; you may want to try taking one of them at a time to see how you feel. You will still be doing something for your health. Remember that small changes make a big difference, as long as they're consistent. Which brings me to my next point: The supplements will always work better in your body than in the bottle, so please remember to take them. Buy yourself a pretty little pillbox you can keep in your go-bag so they'll always be handy. Take them once or twice per day, or as directed in the protocols following.

Last but not least, remember that vitamins alone will not keep you healthy; pleasure and laughter are the greatest nutrients of all. Only these can feed your soul and nourish your spirit! Health plus a negative mind-set equals baditude; health plus a positive outlook equals gratitude!

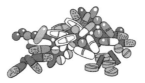

SUPPLEMENTS TO CURE WHAT AILS YOU

This section outlines supplements and offers nutritional suggestions to treat a wide variety of ailments. There's no way I could include every ailment known to (wo)man, so I compiled here the ones I most commonly deal with at my practice. I've listed supplements and dosages, along with advice on what foods are best to treat the problem.

Note: Unless otherwise specified, all supplements should be taken with food. Make sure each of your meals contains some fat to help your body absorb the fat-soluble vitamins A, D, E, and K, as well as CoQ10. Supplements for each ailment are listed in order of importance.

Acne

Supplements:

Zinc	50 mg per day for 3–4 months; then decrease dosage to 25 mg per day for maintenance
Probiotics	8–16 billion organisms per day, in either powdered or capsule form
Vitamin A	25,000 IU for 1 month; then 5,000 IU per day as a maintenance dose. Capsules made from fish oil are quite effective.
Omega-3s	1,000 mg twice per day
Borage oil (GLA)	240 mg twice per day
Vitamin C	500 mg twice per day
Tea tree oil	Apply topically to spot-treat blemishes, 1–2 times per day.

Nutritional Approaches:

This protocol works beautifully for both oily and dry skin types, because the omega-3s and the GLA will regulate your oil production from within. For best results, eliminate sugar, wine, and beer, which will all contribute to breakouts on the skin. Your body will use up its zinc stores just trying to metabolize all the sugar you are eating. Also keep a tight rein on the bread and yeasty foods you eat, which can also worsen the problem. Try to do some yoga once per week for stress management as well.

Allergies (Seasonal or Dietary)

Supplements for seasonal allergies:

Borage oil (GLA)	250 mg twice per day
Omega-3s	1,000 mg twice per day
Quercetin	500 mg twice per day
Astragalus root	200 mg twice per day, in either liquid tincture or tablet form
Echinacea root	100 mg twice per day, in either liquid tincture or tablet form

Supplements for dietary allergies:

You can take the protocol listed above and also add:

L-glutamine	5,000 mg per day in powdered form, mixed into water
Probiotics	8–16 billion organisms per day

Nutritional Approaches:

It's a great idea to eliminate wheat, cheese, and milk, which are three of the most common allergens in our diet today and can exacerbate both food and seasonal allergies. Plain yogurt has numerous health benefits, so if you can tolerate it, go for it! If you can't live without your pasta, try buckwheat (soba) noodles or rice-based cellophane noodles instead; both are sold in the ethnic-foods aisle at the grocery store. Drink plenty of nettle tea, which can also decrease the allergenic response. Quercetin is known for its ability to block the release of histamines, thereby preventing allergy symptoms like swollen nasal passages, congestion, sneezing, watery eyes, and itchiness in eyes and nose.

Bone Health

Supplements:

Vitamin D	1,000 IU per day
Calcium	1,000 mg per day on an empty stomach
Magnesium	400 mg per day on an empty stomach
Omega-3s	1,000 mg per day

You should also take a multivitamin or a trace mineral supplement that contains 25 mg zinc, 2 mg copper, 5 mg boron, and 150 mcg of vitamin K.

Nutritional Approaches:

If there's a history of osteoporosis in your family, get a head start on your bone health right now. It's all about prevention. Get in the habit of weight training 2 or 3 times per week, which is a very important lifestyle habit for building bones. (Weight training has the added benefit of sculpting gorgeously toned muscles.) Also get your vitamin D status checked yearly; your blood test should show a level of 30ng/dl or greater. A diet rich in whole foods that includes adequate protein, sesame seeds or tahini, almonds, and dark green leafy vegetables is imperative. Whether or not you consume dairy, take supplements; a person would have to drink ten tall glasses of vitamin D–fortified milk each day just to get minimum levels of vitamin D into their diet. Also try to get fifteen minutes of sunshine at least three days per week, which will help your body make vitamin D. You must expose as much of your skin as possible without any sunscreen to reap the benefits, because wearing sunscreen with as little as SPF 8 decreases the body's ability to make vitamin D by 95 percent!

Brittle Nails

Supplements:

MSM	1,000 mg three times per day
Calcium	1,000 mg per day
Magnesium	400–800 mg per day
Horsetail	1 teaspoon of liquid extract (2.5 g from *Equisetum arvense* herb) diluted in water or juice

Nutritional Approaches:

Nails are composed of protein, so make sure you eat enough protein each day, as well as essential fatty acids and calcium-rich foods. To pamper your nails, try rubbing olive or coconut oil into the cuticle and nail bed each night. If you have vertical ridges or dark lines down the nails, get your thyroid checked. If you have toenail fungus, try putting tea tree oil directly on top of the nails and under the nail bed. Last but not least, take a break from using nail polish every now and then. Long-term nail polish use can cause dry, brittle nails. Go for the sexy look of naked nails while allowing them to come up for air.

Colds and Flus

Supplements:

Vitamin C	Acute: 250 mg every hour. Maintenance: 500 mg twice per day
Echinacea	Acute: 1 teaspoon (from *Echinacea purpurea* root 2.5 g) three times per day Maintenance: 1 teaspoon 1 or 2 times per day
Olive leaf extract	Two 500 mg capsules three times per day
Maitake D	Two capsules twice per day (two capsules should contain 300 mg maitake mushroom powder and 20 mg maitake standardized extract)
Micellized Vitamin A	For upper-respiratory-tract infections, take 1 dropperful, mixed into a shot of juice, per day for 1 week. For long-term prevention, take 1 dropperful once per week.

Nutritional Approaches:

You know when you've got a cold coming on. Your eyes get a little glassy, your cheeks get flushed, there's a tickle in the back of your throat, your head aches, and you want to crawl right back into bed and sleep until you feel better. The good news is that if you're lucky enough to catch it in time and nip it in the bud, you can prevent a cold from coming on, or at least shorten its duration. Whip out your notebooks and pencils here and start jotting; these nutritional tools will come in handy for the rest of your life. Take the following supplements the minute you feel a cold coming on and for five days after your symptoms are completely resolved, to ensure that you do not have a relapse. Keep them on hand for travel as well. If you were unable to beat your cold to the punch, they will still improve your immune function and may help shorten the duration of your cold, if not the severity.

Echinacea purpurea: Echinacea helps boost the white blood cell count and has natural antiviral properties. The liquid variety is much more effective because it is absorbed much more easily than the tablet form. Gargle with it when you have a sore throat to kill bacteria in the mouth and throat. Make sure you buy a brand with a minimum of 1.0 mg/ml of alkylamides to ensure optimal strength and quality. These substances work together to enhance immune-system function, boost white blood cell count, support respiratory function, and help cleanse the lymphatic system. A good, potent product should temporarily make your tongue feel numb and your mouth salivate; this tells you that active compounds are present.

Drink 8 to 16 ounces of clear liquids every hour. Herbal teas, chicken broth, miso soup, or diluted juices will help flush out the bacteria and mucus from your body. Chop up a whole clove of garlic, add it to a teaspoon of raw honey, and try taking that as well. Suck on zinc lozenges and gargle with diluted echinacea to kill the bacteria in the throat. Eat plenty of orange and dark green vegetables, which are rich sources of Vitamin A.

If your system is really stubborn and these supplements aren't working fast enough to your liking, kick it up a notch and pay a visit to the health-food store. Belly up to the juice counter and order yourself a stiff drink. Freshly juiced vegetable juices (especially chlorophyll-rich green ones) clear out the lymphatic system and have antibacterial benefits, and they'll help you boot out a cold faster than you can say "green goddess"! Try this recipe on for size, either at home or at the juice bar:

WILD WOMEN DO AND THEY DON'T REGRET IT
3 CELERY STALKS
5 LARGE SPINACH LEAVES
2 CARROTS
1 BEET
HANDFUL OF PARSLEY
3-INCH ROUND OF WHEATGRASS

Wash greens thoroughly and put them in the juicer. Juices may be diluted with ½ cup water if desired. You may also add garlic and ginger.

Cold Sores (see Herpes, page 118)

Constipation, Gas, and Bloating

Supplements:

Magnesium	400 mg twice per day on an empty stomach.
Probiotics	8–16 billion organisms per day
Pancreatic enzymes	Take per meal: 160 mg Pancreatin 5X with 20,000 USP units of amylase and protease, and 1,600 USP units of lipase.
Betaine hydrochloride	200 mg per meal
Spanish black radish	1 tablet three times per day

Nutritional Approaches:

Try food-combining principles, which can really lighten the workload of the digestive tract: eat all fruit first thing in the morning, on an empty stomach, half an hour before your breakfast. At meals, combine protein with vegetables and fat or carbohydrates with vegetables and fat, but do not combine protein with carbohydrates. Examples of a meal could be a salad, steak, and sautéed spinach, or beans, brown rice, and veggies. Also make sure to incorporate two to three tablespoons of freshly ground flaxseeds into your oatmeal, yogurt, cottage cheese, or juice. The fiber content in the flaxseeds will help your body make digestive enzymes and will also regulate your bowel movements.

Dandruff

Supplements:

Probiotics	1 capsule (8 billion organisms) twice daily for 1 month; 1 capsule per day for maintenance
Garlic	1 capsule per day; should contain 1 bulb per capsule
Borage oil	Two 240-mg capsules twice daily for 1 month; then 1 capsule twice per day as a maintenance dose
Spanish black radish	1 capsule three times per day

Nutritional Approaches:

Dandruff is often an indication that your system contains a high amount of yeast, so limit your intake of sugar, yeasted foods, and foods that have trace amounts of fungus or mold (pasta, bread, cheese, sweets, mushrooms, soy sauce, vinegar, wine, and peanuts).

Depression

Supplements:

Omega-3s	6,000–9,000 mg per day, with meals, in either liquid or capsule form
Inositol	Start with 1 teaspoon mixed in water three times per day. For severe depression, take 2 teaspoons three times daily.
Folic acid	2 mg per day
St. John's wort *or*	1 teaspoon of liquid tincture (from *Hypericum perforatum* flowering herb 2.5 g) at bedtime
5-HTP	300 mg per day

Nutritional Approaches:

Depression is often associated with insulin resistance, so watch out for too many sugars, even if you crave them. Try to get a balance of protein, healthy fats, and complex carbohydrates at each meal to offset cravings and stabilize your blood sugar. Make sure you get your rear in gear and head to the gym for at least thirty minutes per day. Exercise is nature's antidepressant; it naturally raises your serotonin levels. Also make sure you get some fresh air and sunlight on a daily basis, which helps with hormonal regulation. Never take St. John's wort with 5-HTP, as it can cause serotonin syndrome, a potentially lethal syndrome caused by a combination or two or more drugs that raise serotonin levels to toxic levels; either take St. John's Wort *or* 5 HTP.

Diarrhea

Supplements:

L-glutamine powder	1 teaspoon mixed into water every 3 hours
Probiotics	1 capsule or 1 teaspoon powder (8 billion organisms) every 3 hours
Omega-3s	1,000–2,000 mg per day
Boswellia extract	300 mg two to four times per day

Nutritional Approaches:
Try the BRATT diet: bananas, white rice, applesauce, tea, and toast. These will all help bind you up and slow down the pace of your intestinal spasm. Also beef up your fiber intake with two to three tablespoons of ground flaxseeds each day. If you have colitis, IBS, Crohn's disease, or a more serious condition, visit www.scdiet.org and www.scdiet.com for incredible nutritional support with a gluten-free diet.

Dry Skin

Supplements:

Evening primrose oil	3,000 mg per day
Omega-3s	2,000 mg per day

Nutritional Approaches:
Add flaxseed oil liberally to salads to act as an internal moisturizer. Make sure you bathe in warm, not hot, water so you don't overdry your skin. Keep coconut or olive oil in a spray bottle and apply it to damp skin after a shower. These oils are rich in natural emollients and will lock in moisture. A good rule of thumb is that if you won't eat it, don't put it on your skin! Also make sure to get your thyroid checked out; dry skin can be a sign of an underactive

thyroid. Use a humidifier (or even a pan of water placed near a radiator) to humidify your environment, especially in winter. This helps to reduce the amount of moisture lost from the skin through evaporation.

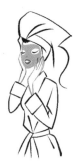

BEAUTY MASK FOR DRY SKIN

1 EGG

1 TEASPOON HONEY

1/2 TEASPOON OLIVE OIL

A FEW DROPS OF ROSEWATER

Mix the ingredients thoroughly and use as a mask. Leave on for 10 minutes and rinse off with warm water. Gently pat your skin dry and apply moisturizer if needed.

Fibrocystic Breasts

Supplements:

DIM	200 mg per day
Chaste tree	4 tablets per day (from *Vitex agnus-castus* fruit; 500mg). *Note:* Do *not* take chaste tree if you are on the pill.
Evening primrose oil	2,000 mg per day
Milk thistle	150 mg twice per day
Spanish black radish	1 tablet with meals

Nutritional Approaches:

The best thing you can do for painful breasts is to clear caffeine from your diet. Caffeine can greatly influence premenstrual breast tenderness. Drink plenty of water and limit high-salt foods so your breasts won't feel like two watermelons attached to your torso. Add two to three tablespoons of ground flaxseeds to your daily diet by tossing them into your oatmeal, yogurt, cottage cheese, salads, or a protein smoothie. After your period is finished each month, give yourself a breast self-examination, so you know your own lumpiness. Better yet, have your partner do it, which can be much more fun!

Hangovers

Supplements the night before:

Milk thistle	300 mg
Schisandra	1 teaspoon of liquid tincture (250 mg)
DMAE	200 mg
Vitamin B_1	50 mg

Supplements the morning after:

Magnesium	400 mg as a rescue remedy
N-acetyl cysteine	1,000 mg
MSM	Start by taking 1,500 mg. After an hour, feel free to add another 1,500 mg if you need extra support.
L-glutamine	5,000 mg of powder dissolved in water for a sour stomach

Nutritional Approaches:

Make sure you eat while you drink; drinking on an empty stomach is a fast ride on the expressway to a hangover. (Please refer back to Chapter 3, "Drinking Gorgeous," for a more in-depth discussion.) Fight alcohol-induced dehydration by alternating boozy cocktails with glasses of water or club soda with lemon. Take a disco nap before you head out for a night on the town, and get plenty of rest the next day. Drink tomato juice and eat crackers with raw honey the morning after to help your body metabolize the alcohol in your system.

Herpes

Supplements:

Olive leaf extract	2,000 mg every 3 hours
L-lysine	3,000 mg capsules twice per day
Vitamin C	1,000 mg three times per day
Calcium lactate	250 mg twice per day
St. John's wort	(from *Hypericum perforatum* flowering herb 2.5 g) 1 teaspoon diluted in a shot of water or juice
Echinacea	(from *Echinacea purpurea* root 1:2 extract) 1 teaspoon diluted in a shot of water or juice

Nutritional Approaches:

Steer clear of nuts and nut butters, as well as all soy products. These foods are very high in arginine, which can exacerbate a herpes outbreak. Also be careful of excess alcohol and sugar, which can suppress the immune system.

High Cortisol Levels

Supplements:

Omega-3s	1,000 mg twice per day
Phosphatidylserine	300 mg at bedtime
Licorice root	(from *Glycyrrhiza glabra* root 2.5 g) First thing in the morning, take 1 teaspoonful of liquid tincture diluted in an ounce of water
Ashwagandha root	First thing in the morning, take 1 teaspoonful of liquid tincture from *Withania somnifera* root 2.5 gm diluted in an ounce of water

Nutritional Approaches:

Have your doctor check your DHEA (dehydroepiandrosterone) levels. DHEA is a hormone that is made by the adrenal glands and is easily converted into other hormones, especially estrogen and testosterone. Low DHEA can cause hormonal and sleep disturbances, and high cortisol often lowers DHEA. Now is the time to try some deep breathing and relaxation techniques, which will also lower your cortisol levels. The same goes for yoga; even ten minutes a day will help lower your cortisol levels.

Insomnia and Poor Sleep

Supplements:

L-theanine	200 mg one hour before bedtime
GABA	550 mg one hour before bedtime
5-HTP	300 mg per day

Nutritional Approaches:
Avoid sugar and alcohol before bed, as they cause fluctuations in your blood sugar levels and, ultimately, disrupt your sleep. Also check in with yourself about that caffeine habit of yours; even one cup of coffee in the morning can affect your sleep cycle that evening. A couple of hours before bed, eat a snack consisting of protein and some fruit; this combination will help your body make serotonin and melatonin, which should keep you slumbering all night. Sleep tight!

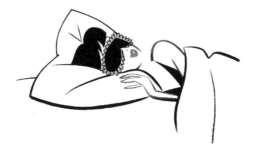

Low Energy

Supplements:

Licorice root	(from *Glycyrrhiza glabra* root 2.5 g) First thing in the morning, take 1 teaspoonful of liquid tincture diluted in an ounce of water
Ashwagandha root	First thing in the morning, take 1 teaspoonful of liquid tincture from *Withania somnifera* root 2.5 g diluted in an ounce of water
L-carnitine	1,000 mg three times per day
Magnesium	400 mg twice per day
Lipoic acid	300 mg per day
CoQ10	100 mg twice per day

Nutritional Approaches:

First and foremost, get your thyroid and mercury levels checked to rule out any organic causes. Check in with yourself and see what environmental stressors could be causing you to feel wiped out. Scoot on over to your fave yoga studio and get busy with some sun salutations and downward dogs. You'll be amazed at your energy levels afterward! Also keep your caffeine intake to a minimum; it will only give you a temporary energy fix.

Menstrual Cramps

Supplements:

Cramp bark	1 teaspoon liquid tincture diluted in juice (from *Viburnum opulus* bark 2.5 g). Begin taking it the week before your period, and continue during your period as needed.
Magnesium	400 mg twice per day
Calcium lactate	250 mg every 3 hours while cramps are active
Evening primrose oil	3,000 mg per day

Nutritional Approaches:

Eat three to four ounces of protein at each meal, especially the week before your period. Protein supports liver function and will help your body metabolize your hormones. Steer clear of any and all hydrogenated oils, which can generate severe inflammation that will aggravate menstrual cramps. Also look out for too much booze, which can temporarily alleviate cramps but will worsen them when the alcohol has worn off. If you need to take anti-inflammatory drugs for the pain, also take a heaping teaspoon of L-glutamine powder with water to avoid irritating the lining of your stomach.

Mercury Toxicity

Supplements:

Spanish black radish	1 tablet three times per day
Phosphatidylcholine	1,000 mg twice per day
Lipoic acid	300 mg per day
Omega-3s	1,000 mg twice per day
Aqueous selenium	400 mcg per day
Probiotics	16 billion organisms per day
Garlic	1 capsule per day; should contain 1 bulb per capsule
MSM	2,000 mg per day

Nutritional Approaches:

Work with a nutritionally oriented physician to get your mercury levels checked. If your levels are high, it might be necessary to undergo chelation therapy. It is helpful to monitor your levels on an annual basis. Cook with cilantro, which naturally chelates mercury. Try it as a base for pesto sauce. Try to eat as cleanly as possible, with plenty of protein, whole grains, and dark green leafy vegetables, which will give your body the support it needs to eliminate mercury. Incorporate wild Alaskan salmon, sardines, and halibut (from www.vitalchoice.com) into your diet as a clean source of fish. Also check out Chapter 2, "Eating Gorgeous," and Chapter 7, "Gorgeous Questions and Answers," for a more comprehensive discussion on mercury in fish.

PMS

Supplements:

Milk thistle	300 mg per day
Calcium	500 mg twice per day on an empty stomach
Magnesium	400–800 mg on an empty stomach
Inositol	1 teaspoon of powder mixed into water, up to 6 times per day
St. John's wort	1 teaspoon of liquid tincture (from *Hypericum perforatum* flowering herb 2.5 g)
Omega-3s	2,000 mg per day
Borage oil	500 mg per day

Nutritional Approaches:

As with menstrual cramps, make sure you are eating enough protein and dark green, leafy vegetables throughout the day, especially the week before your period. Be mindful of St. John's wort if you take the pill; about 1 percent of the population has a decrease in contraceptive efficacy. For bad PMS that has you on edge, plunk yourself down in an Epsom salts bath and soak away your stress! Also hustle on over to a yoga class, or pop in a yoga DVD at home. Yoga does wonders for leveling out your hormones.

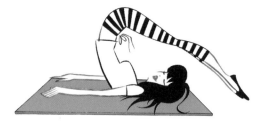

Polycystic Ovarian Syndrome

Supplements:

Chromium picolinate	500 mcg twice per day
Lipoic acid	300 mg twice per day
Omega-3s	3,000 mg per day
Evening primrose oil	1,000 mg per day
Vitamin D	1,000 IU per day

Nutritional Approaches:
PCOS is linked to insulin resistance, so look out for sugar. Try to eat as balanced a diet as you can, and trade in sugary sodas for flavored seltzers. Try sweetening your foods with agave syrup or stevia powder, both of which are naturally low in sugar and chemical-free.

Quitting Smoking

Supplements:

Licorice root	(from *Glycyrrhiza glabra* root 2.5 g) First thing in the morning, take 1 teaspoonful of liquid tincture diluted in an ounce of water
Tyrosine	1,000 mg per day
5-HTP	100 mg per day
Vitamin C	500 mg three times per day
B-complex vitamins	50 mg per day

Nutritional Approaches:
When you initially quit smoking, you may find that you crave sugar like crazy, because your blood sugar will be all over the road map for the first few months. To help your body adjust, try adding green vegetable juices to your diet a few times per week. They will pump your insides with hundreds of vitamins and minerals and help your lungs and adrenal glands heal and recover, which will ultimately stabilize your mood and your cravings. Also try keeping a bottle of lavender essential oil handy; a few dabs on your wrist a few times a day will help promote relaxation.

Sugar Cravings

Supplements:

Lipoic acid	300 mg per day
Calcium	500 mg twice per day
Magnesium	400 mg twice per day
Zinc	25 mg per day
Aqueous selenium	200 mcg per day
Tyrosine	500 mg twice per day on an empty stomach; you can take up to 2,000 mg per day if needed.
5-HTP	300 mg per day
L-glutamine	5,000 mg per day in powdered form, mixed into water

Nutritional Approaches:

It can take your body up to seven days to eliminate sugar from your system, so try to go without it cold turkey. (Once you're over the hump, it does get easier, I promise!) It's very important to eat small, frequent meals throughout the day to stabilize your blood sugar. Snack on raw nuts and seeds, which are rich in trace minerals that will help curb cravings. Also avoid diet sodas and artificial sweeteners and allow some time for your taste buds to learn a new way of living; you're better off using agave syrup or stevia powder, or even a little maple syrup or honey.

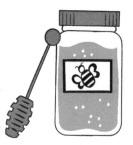

Thinning Hair

Supplements:

Zinc	25 mg per day
Magnesium	400 mg per day
Hyaluronic acid	150 mg per day
N-acetyl cysteine	1,000 mg per day
Omega-3s	2,000 mg per day
Evening primrose oil	1,000 mg per day

Nutritional Approaches:

Chicken stock made from bones is naturally rich in hyaluronic acid, and root vegetables like sweet potatoes are naturally rich in magnesium, so feel free to incorporate both into your diet. Your local health-food store is a valuable resource for premade organic chicken stock, and I like to cook brown rice in the stock for a yummy risotto. Medically, make sure you get your thyroid checked; an under- or overactive thyroid can be a cause for thinning hair. In addition, stress can cause hair loss, so take a minute to reflect on what's been happening in your life in the past six months or so.

Thyroid

BMR Test (Basal Metabolic Rate Test)

This test (page 126) is an excellent way to determine your thyroid function using your basal body temperature, or your body's temperature at rest. My clients often come in with normal lab values on a thyroid test, yet when they take their BMR test it is low, indicating sluggish thyroid function. If the thyroid is running low, the body's temperature will drop below normal while you're at rest or asleep.

The test is done by measuring your underarm temperature upon waking after a night's sleep. For accuracy, the test is performed five mornings in a row, and then the average is calculated. It's critical that you do not perform this test during ovulation (usually days 11 through 14 of your monthly cycle), because your body temperature may be falsely elevated during that time.

Instructions for the test:

1. The night before, shake down an oral glass thermometer and set it in a safe place next to the bed.

2. Immediately upon waking, without raising your head from the pillow, place the thermometer in one armpit.

3. Leave the thermometer under your arm for ten minutes.

4. Move as little as possible during the process and try to remain flat on your back. Otherwise the thyroid gland will be activated and a false reading will be taken.

5. After ten minutes, remove the thermometer and record the temperature.

A temperature of between 97.8 and 98.2 degrees is considered normal. If you fall below the normal range, please scoot on over to your nutritionally oriented doctor's office for further guidance.

Urinary Tract Infections (UTIs)

Supplements:

D-mannose

Day 1 of an active UTI: ½ level teaspoon (1 gram of D-mannose) mixed into 6 ounces of water every 2 hours, 8 A.M.–8 P.M.

Day 2: ½ level teaspoon mixed into 6 ounces of water every 3 hours, 8 A.M.–8 P.M.

Day 3: ½ level teaspoon mixed into 6 ounces of water every 4 hours, 8 A.M.–8 P.M.

For maintenance: take ½ teaspoon daily mixed into 6 ounces of water.

For preventing "honeymoon cystitis," take 1 teaspoonful of powder one hour prior to boom-boom and then again immediately afterward.

Vitamin C

1,000 mg per day. Use the ascorbic acid form of vitamin C, which can help acidify the urine and discourage bacterial growth.

Probiotics

8–16 billion organisms per day, in either powdered or capsule form with meals.

Nutritional Approaches:

Cranberry products are well known for their incredible capacity to fight UTIs. In addition to acidifying the urine, cranberries contain substances that inhibit bacteria from attaching to the bladder lining and, ultimately, promote the flushing out of bacteria with the urine stream. Here's the catch: sugar will feed the bacteria that cause UTIs, so use only lip-puckering, unsweetened cranberry juice, cranberry extract capsules, or naturally sweet blueberries, which contain similar UTI-fighting substances. I like to dilute unsweetened cranberry juice in water for a refreshingly tart drink. Epicatechin, a bioflavonoid found in both cranberries and blueberries, is also believed to inhibit the attachment of the bacteria to the lining of the bladder.

Vaginal Dryness

Supplements:

Wheat-germ oil:	Insert a capsule into the vagina at bedtime
Evening primrose oil:	1 capsule twice daily
Omega-3s:	2 capsules twice daily

Nutritional Approaches:

Eat a healthy, whole-foods diet rich in nutrients and trace minerals, as well as essential fatty acids. Go through your cabinets and clean out the junk fats that will disrupt your body's delicate fatty acid balance: hydrogenated oils, palm oil, vegetable oil, soybean oil, margarine, and Crisco. Instead, stock your refrigerator with flaxseed oil and flaxseeds, wild Alaskan salmon, organic olive oil, coconut oil, walnut oil, and raw nuts and seeds. These will keep you moisturized and lubricated from the inside out. Don't forget to work with a nutritionally oriented physician to get your DHEA, estrogen, and progesterone levels checked, since hormonal imbalances could also be an underlying cause of vaginal dryness.

Water Retention

Supplements:

Vitamin B$_6$	50 mg twice per day
Taurine	1,000 mg twice per day
Horsetail	1 teaspoon of liquid extract (2.5 g from *Equisetum arvense* herb) diluted in water or juice

Nutritional Approaches:

Drink dandelion tea throughout the day for gentle diuretic benefits. Unsweetened cranberry juice diluted in water also provides diuretic benefits, as does eating asparagus, watermelon, and freshly steamed or sautéed dandelion greens.

Workout Recovery

Supplements:

Calcium	500 mg before each workout and 500 mg before bedtime
Magnesium	400 mg before each workout and 400 mg before bedtime
CoQ10	100 mg before each workout
Lipoic acid	100 mg before and after each workout
L-carnitine	1,000 mg first thing in the morning and 1,000 mg after each workout. Try to take all L-carnitine before 4:00 P.M.
Omega-3s	1,000 mg twice per day

Nutritional Approaches:

Within an hour after working out, eat a meal that combines protein, carbo-hydrates, and fats to replace your glycogen stores and balance your blood sugar. If you feel like you might be sore the next day, plunk yourself down in a warm Epsom salts bath for twenty minutes. Two cups of salts per bath should do the trick.

If you're training for an endurance event, make your own healthy sports repletion drink: 8 ounces of organic juice, such as apple, grape, or pomegranate, mixed with 8 ounces water and $1/8$ teaspoon sea salt. Combine all the ingredients and shake well. This can be stored for up to twenty-four hours in the refrigerator. You can also make your own power gel—take 2 tablespoons of raw, organic honey and add one of the following: 2 tablespoons raw peanut butter, 2 tablespoons apple butter, or half a banana. Combine the ingredients and run through the blender until smooth and creamy. Add 1 teaspoon lemon juice (to cut the sweetness) and blend again. This can be carried during a long run in a fuel-belt bottle, available in sports stores or running shops.

Yeast and Sinus Infections

Supplements:

Probiotics	8 billion organisms twice per day
Garlic	1 capsule twice per day; should contain 1 bulb per capsule
Spanish black radish	1 tablet per meal
Boric acid suppositories	600 mg boric acid suppositories inserted vaginally every night before bed for three to five nights

Nutritional Approaches:

Cook with fresh garlic and coconut oil, which are natural antifungals that fight yeast. Limit your intake of sugar and sweets, yeasted foods, and foods that have trace amounts of fungus or mold (pasta, bread, sweets, mushrooms, soy sauce, vinegar, wine, and peanuts). Look out for the yeastier alcoholic drinks like wine and beer; stick to hard alcohols with a splash of club soda and lime.

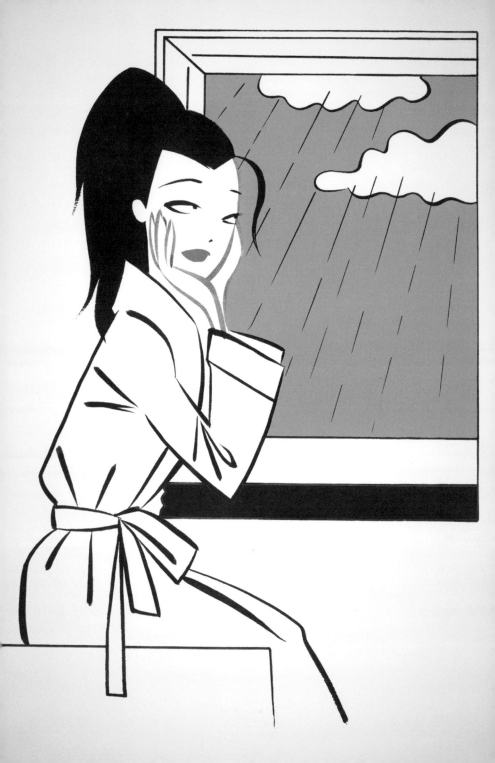

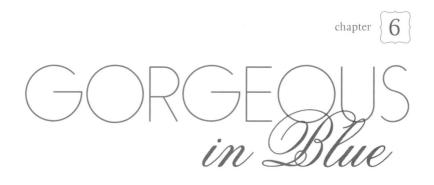

chapter 6

GORGEOUS in Blue

A woman is like a tea bag—you never know how strong she is until she gets in hot water. —Eleanor Roosevelt

Let's face it, babes, we've all been down in the dumps at one time or another. We've all had days, weeks, or even months where we felt crummy due to those all too familiar problems: PMS, depression, or a bad breakup. This chapter is great to flip to when you're feeling blue and you need a little divine intervention. Wipe your tears. Help is on the way!

In this chapter, I'll offer tips on how to cope with a variety of afflictions that can affect us at any point in our lives. Don't worry, I'm not going to chastise you for drowning your sorrows in a bowl of pudding. And I'm not going to prescribe seaweed and bulgur to cure a broken heart. Instead, I'm going to offer some moral support, some advice on how to eat well for comfort, and I'm going to give you the goods on keeping your moods level. Tough experiences certainly aren't fun to go through, but if you can ride them out and learn something, they're often worth the journey.

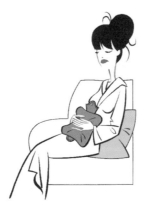

PMS: YOU'VE GOT TO GO WITH THE FLOW

How do you know when you've got premenstrual syndrome? When you're screeching at the poor cashier at the deli for being out of Snickers, that's usually a good indication. Other side effects include moodiness (often it's our friends and significant others who bear the brunt of this), bloating, breasts that feel like water balloons, breakouts that resemble mini constellations, fatigue, and sometimes even cramping (and this is even before your period has started!). The average woman in the United States menstruates 480 times in a lifetime; that means 480 potential bouts of PMS. Oh, the joys of womanhood!

I'm happy to report that you can make PMS a thing of the past, or at the very least you can greatly curb it. I'm going to help you get to the root of your problem by correcting the major causes of PMS: hormonal imbalances, low blood sugar, poor liver detoxification, and an imbalance of nutrients. Follow my program and you can expect to see results in as little as one cycle. So come on, princess, wipe that pretty little pout off your face! A few posh pills and some wellness guidelines will put you back in top form.

PMS Eradication Plan

The first step in bidding adieu to PMS is to eat your protein. Protein supports the liver, which detoxifies estrogen as it fluctuates through your system. Plus, it balances your hormones and stabilizes your blood sugar. So make sure that you eat adequate amounts of protein throughout the day and throughout your cycle. At least two out of three meals per day should contain three or more ounces of protein, such as lean meats, poultry, eggs, or fish. This protein will help balance your blood sugar and prevent mood swings during times of stress. If you're cooking, an easy way to measure protein is by resting the portion in the palm of your hand; a four-ounce serving of protein should fit easily into your palm. One egg counts as one ounce of protein.

Next, eliminate or minimize caffeinated and chemical-laden beverages such as diet sodas, coffee, and black tea, and flush your body with filtered water and antioxidant-rich green or white teas. Here's a Gorgeous Girl mocktail that won't steer you wrong: Try brewing two bags of green tea with one bag of peppermint tea in a large pitcher. Toss in two tablespoons of agave syrup or honey to lace the tea with sweetness. Steep the bags for one hour, then remove them and refrigerate the tea. *Voilà*—your very own antioxidant-rich bevvie! Drink it straight up throughout the day, or use it as a mixer for green tea-tinis. Now, don't go hog wild and drink twenty glasses of tea—one or two will do you justice. The rest of your liquid intake really does need to come from water to keep you hydrated and energized; six to eight glasses per day are the general rule of thumb (see pages 59–61 for more information on hydration).

Prevention is key when it comes to curtailing PMS. Eat healthfully all month long to enable your body to truly regulate itself, its hormones, and its blood sugar, and to provide good liver support (for more detail see Chapter 2, "Eating Gorgeous"). Do yourself a favor and cut out all sugary foods, white flour, artificial sweeteners, margarine, and fried or processed foods. I know, I know, girls—ouch! Nobody said it would be easy, but there's no way around it.

Why should Gorgeous Girls avoid margarine, hydrogenated and partially hydrogenated vegetable oils, and fried foods? Margarine and fried foods are first-rate drivers in the toxic-fats Grand Prix. Margarine is a man-made substance that is pure poison. Not only does it gum up the insides of your arteries, but it also depletes your reserves of good fats. Margarine is produced by bombarding vegetable oil with hydrogen molecules until it converts into a solid form. At the molecular level, the structure of margarine is not found in nature, so the body has a very hard time recognizing what it is and therefore can't break it down. What that means for you is a total disruption of hormones and fatty acids, prompting menstrual cramps, breast tenderness, headaches, and a host of other symptoms. (Whereas good fats can help keep all of these symptoms in check.) At the end of the day, I don't care if it's trans fat–free margarine, soy margarine, or bird-turd margarine. If it's a Franken-fat of any form, avoid it! Only the finest, purest, most natural fats will fight PMS.

Same goes for artificial sweeteners. These can wreak just as much havoc on your blood sugar as regular table sugar. The sweet taste tricks your brain into believing that it's eaten something sweet, prompting the same rise in blood sugar as regular sugar would, which can promote weight gain. And it gets worse: Artificial sweeteners also interfere with the uptake of serotonin and dopamine in the brain—two neurotransmitters that give us a happy, contented feeling. Ultimately, artificial sweeteners can cause or worsen depression. Who needs that? Luckily, the gods have smiled on us and have given us two options for our sweet tooth. One is stevia powder. The stevia plant is remarkably sweet and has no calories. Use it sparingly, as a little goes a very long way. The other is agave syrup, which tastes and looks a lot like honey and has much less sugar. You'll find both at your local health-food store.

MAKING PMS A THING OF THE PAST

- Look out for processed foods, excess sugar, and caffeine—these will tip the scales for mood swings, cravings, and irritability.

- Eat meals and snacks throughout the day, and make sure you get some protein in at each meal.

- Try taking supplements to curb your PMS: milk thistle, calcium, magnesium, GLA, and omega-3s for starters.

- If at first you don't succeed, try and try again: Add in inositol and St. John's wort for really stubborn mood swings associated with PMS.

- Be mindful of St. John's wort if you take the pill: about 1 percent of the population has a decrease in contraceptive efficacy.

In addition to choosing the right foods, it helps to take supplements that will give your body the vitamins and minerals it needs to prevent prostaglandin production (prostaglandins are short-lived hormones that can create the cramping associated with PMS). Your hormones, especially estrogen, are detoxified by the liver into less carcinogenic forms. Support your liver with milk thistle, also known by the herbal peeps as silymarin. A dose of 150 mg per day will do wonders to lighten your flow and shorten the duration of your period, as well as support and detoxify your liver all month long. This means balanced hormonal function and a greater feeling of well-being and energy on a consistent basis.

To regulate your moods, calcium and magnesium are a girl's best friend. These trace minerals will really chill you out. Not only do they fight PMS, but they also relieve menstrual cramping by helping your muscles relax, which enables the uterine muscles to relax. Ultimately, all this relaxation is going to have a calming effect on your mood, too. So don't even think of running out of these precious minerals when "Flo" is in town. Have you ever noticed that you crave chocolate before your period? It's no surprise, given that chocolate is very rich in magnesium. So if you're craving chocolate, try supplementing with magnesium first—it should do the trick! A good rule of thumb is approximately a 2:1 ratio of calcium to magnesium: 1,000 mg of calcium and 400 mg of magnesium per day. Feel free to go up to 800 mg of magnesium per day if you suffer from stubborn constipation or while you're having bad cramps. And make sure you snack on raw nuts and seeds and have dark, leafy greens one or two times per day to get in your dietary supply of these trace minerals. You can also eat a couple squares of dark chocolate for a delicious boost of magnesium that's both naughty and nice.

Don't forget that the right fats are our friends, not our foes. Two fats you'll want to get in are GLA (gamma linoleic acid; 240 mg per day), and the omega-3 rock stars EPA and DHA (1,000 mg per day). These fats will fight the production of prostaglandins, stabilize your blood sugar and your mood, and, as an added perk, keep your skin supple and soft. If you have severe depression-related PMS or suffer from depression year-round, you can increase your dosage of EPA and DHA to 3,000–6,000 mg per day, as a therapeutic dose. Fish oils are pretty incredible: They raise serotonin levels in the brain and have been clinically proven to fight depression. Best part yet, they will not interfere with antidepressants—though if you are indeed on antidepressants, you should always run any supplements by your physician or psychopharmacologist first. Dietwise, make sure you're eating plenty of wild-caught fish, which contain a much greater amount of omega-3s than their farm-raised counterparts. Grass-fed beef is another rich source of omega-3s that should be incorporated into your diet if possible. You'll find it at Whole Foods and www.grassfedbeef.org.

Okay, you say, you've tried all these options and you're still a witchy woman. Not to fear, my dear—we're not at the end of our rope yet! Let's talk for a minute about inositol powder. Inositol is a B vitamin that really takes the edge off your mood and calms you right down. When my pappy had his heart surgery, I downed the stuff like Pixy Stix. Inositol supports liver function, normalizes your hormones, combats insomnia, fights polycystic ovarian syndrome, and helps with depression and obsessive-compulsive disorder. You can take it on an as-needed basis (i.e., the week before your period) or all month long, for optimal results. It tastes slightly sweet and gritty; mix it into water or juice. Inositol can be taken either with food or on an empty stomach. I tell my patients to start off with one teaspoon per day before bedtime or anytime they are feeling edgy. If you'd like to increase your dose, you can build up to six teaspoons per day, though for most people one or two teaspoons per day will suffice. Inositol will not interfere with most antidepressant medications, though it is imperative that you check with your doctor first. Potential side effects may include a few days of gas and diarrhea, though I have not seen this in my practice.

St. John's wort is another powerful remedy that helps control depression and takes the edge off any witchiness that may be creeping in. Now, I know that my herbalist gal pals often take some heat for doling out the stuff on a regular basis ("Dude, don't drink the juice, man"), but used properly, St. John's has its place. St. John's is a nervine that has mildly sedative effects. One teaspoon of liquid extract before bed (you can take it with inositol) will help you sleep peacefully and calmly; but if you're facing a nerve-wracking

MENAGE À TROIS

If you've checked into the heartbreak hotel, you may find you're ready to try your first threesome: you, Ben, and Jerry. You hop into bed in your beat-up sweats with a pint of Chunky Monkey and a spoon. You pull the lid open, peel off the plastic wrap, and slide your spoon into the creamy, rich, ice-cold heaven. You close your eyes and hear pleasure-filled moans fill the room. Faster than you realize, it's all gone. Was it worth it? For the time being, absolutely. But if this becomes your nightly ritual, fast will come the time when you can no longer fit into your favorite jeans, and the honeymoon phase of creamy lust will end—along with your prior enchantment of a threesome.

day of work ahead, then by all means take it in the morning! St. John's wort also has antiviral properties. Considering that 1 in 4 people in the world has genital herpes, and that the surge in premenstrual hormones can cause a flare-up of symptoms, wouldn't you want to take St. John's wort and kill two birds with one stone? I thought so. But if you're still not convinced, pay a visit to your local sassy holistic nutritionist for more information on this wonderfully potent and effective herb.

A GORGEOUS GUIDE TO SURVIVING A BREAKUP

Is there anything worse than a breakup? The answer to that is no—unless, of course, you're sorry that you didn't do it sooner! Whether you're crying over your losses or crying with joy at your newfound freedom, breakups can wreak havoc on your mood and health.

If you are the dumper, you may carry guilt over hurting your honey's feelings. You may have been filled with dread the days, weeks, or even months before the breakup. When you finally do cut the cord, you may need to run for cover from the hot anger headed your way. Or you might be angry with yourself for the way you handled the whole process. If you're the dumpee, you may need to run *under* your covers to seek comfort, indulge in long calls to friends, watch sad movies, and cry your eyes out. It's never easy or fun, but the period of days and weeks post-breakup is the ideal time to

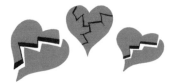

reflect on what we liked and disliked about the person and the relationship itself. You may also want to think about what was good inside the relationship (sex), and what needed work (everything else).

When your world has been rocked by the end of a relationship, how do you put your best foot forward and help yourself feel gorgeous when you don't feel your best? You may feel like you're going through the motions for a while, but go through them anyway. Over time, you'll remember what you used to enjoy doing before you were involved in a relationship, and you'll get your single groove back. Eventually joy and pleasure in everyday activities will feel authentic again, I promise you! So let's pull out our bag of coping tricks and see what lies in store for you on the road to recovery.

Getting Comfortable with Comfort Foods

When you've gone through a breakup, it's okay to slacken the rules a bit and indulge your cravings. It won't last forever, and you'll ride it out. While some women lose their appetite after a breakup, the rest of us find ourselves facedown in a trough of mashed potatoes, sour cream stuck to our chins. Reason being: Eating high-fat, high-sugar foods is a form of self-medication. It temporarily triggers the brain's production of serotonin, making you comfortably numb during this most traumatic time.

But does a breakup mean you should go on a high-fat, sugary food bender? Absolutely not, dollface! I've listed the real-deal comfort foods and some healthier versions to try so you can make some informed choices. And although I don't typically advocate eating low-fat foods all the time, in some cases you can make healthy substitutions without sacrificing the taste you're looking for. Let's make post-breakup weight gain a thing of the past! With a little effort and planning, you can have your cake and eat it too.

Splurge: Ice Cream

A half cup of Ben & Jerry's averages out at 300 calories and 17 grams of fat, depending on the flavor you choose. This means that if you binge on the whole pint, you've just ingested 1,200 calories from ice cream at one sitting, and 68 grams of fat! To put this into perspective for you, that's more than a Whopper with cheese, which clocks in at 680 calories and 39 grams of fat.

Solution: Sorbet

A half cup of most sorbets checks out at 110 calories, 27 grams of sugar, and 0 grams of fat. Cold comfort, here I come!

Splurge: Spaghetti

Most people eat two cups of cooked pasta on average, which has 400 calories and a whopping 80 grams of carbohydrates; that's more than twice the amount of carbs found in an 8-ounce glass of regular soda. Yikes! We haven't even covered the sauces yet (tomato sauce has 90 calories per cup; vodka sauce has 380 calories per cup), or the meat (another 200 calories per 3 ounces) and Parmesan cheese that goes on top (50 calories for 2 tablespoons).

Solution: Soba Noodles

Buck up your mood and the nutrient content by switching over to soba noodles, which are made from buckwheat. Two cups of cooked soba noodles contains 220 calories, 48 grams of carbohydrates, and 12 grams of protein. These are delicious tossed with pesto sauce and stir-fried vegetables.

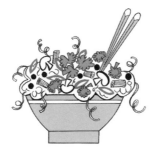

Splurge: Mac and Cheese

Loaded with cheese, butter, and whole milk, this pasta dish quickly turns into a diet disaster at 508 calories and 26 grams of fat per serving.

Solution: Mac and Cheese Makeover

I found a recipe makeover for a healthier mac and cheese at www.foodfit.com:

2 TABLESPOONS OLIVE OIL
2 TABLESPOONS ALL-PURPOSE FLOUR
1 1/2 CUPS NONFAT MILK, HOT, BUT NOT BOILING
1/2 CUP FRESHLY GRATED PARMESAN CHEESE
SALT AND FRESHLY GROUND BLACK PEPPER
3/4 POUND MACARONI NOODLES
1/4 CUP GRATED SHARP CHEDDAR CHEESE
1/4 CUP BREAD CRUMBS

1. Preheat the oven to 375 degrees F and lightly brush a 2-quart casserole dish with olive oil.

2. Bring a large pot of salted water to a boil.

3. In a 2-quart saucepan, whisk the 2 tablespons olive oil and flour together over medium heat. Cook until the mixture gives off a "nutty" aroma, about 2 minutes. Slowly whisk in the hot milk and simmer, stirring occasionally, for 5 minutes. Stir in the Parmesan cheese and season with salt and pepper. Set aside.

4. Add the macaroni to the boiling water and cook until the pasta is al dente, about 7 or 8 minutes. Drain the pasta.

5. Pour the macaroni into the prepared casserole dish. Immediately pour the milk mixture over it and stir to combine. Sprinkle the grated cheddar cheese over the top and then sprinkle the bread crumbs over the cheese.

6. Bake, uncovered, for about 30 minutes, or until the edges are bubbling and the top is golden brown. Remove from the oven and let stand for 10 minutes before serving.

Serving size: 1½ cups

Calories: 367. Total fat: 10 g, saturated fat: 4 g, protein: 17 g, total carbohydrates: 51 g, cholesterol: 13 mg, dietary fiber: 2 g.

Splurge: Mashed Potatoes

Considering that a serving of mashed potatoes can have up to 300 calories (gulp!), I had to come up with another option so I could keep my girlish figure—and still enjoy the best of the comfort foods.

Solution: Mashed Cauliflower

Cruciferous cauliflower to the rescue! It's oh so healthful and delicious, no one (including you) will know the difference between these guys and whipped potatoes. Take 1 head of cauliflower and chop it up into florets. Throw it in a 2-quart stockpot; add in 1 cup of chicken broth and cover. Steam the cauliflower on medium heat for 20 minutes, or until fork-tender. Add more broth if necessary. Pour the cooked cauliflower and broth into a blender; add 1/4 cup olive oil and 1/2 teaspoon sea salt. Blend to desired consistency: less time for a chunkier texture, more for a creamier one. Mmmmmm! Serves 4; 70 calories per serving.

Splurge: Salt-and-Vinegar Potato Chips

A 1.5-ounce bag has 210 calories, half of which come from fat. And believe you me, it's not from organic olive oil, either. Also bear in mind that the potatoes used to make chips are the supermarket rejects that neither you nor I would bring home for dinner.

Solution: Salted Air-Popped Popcorn

Packed with fiber and low in calories, air-popped popcorn gives you far more bang for your buck: 1 cup has 31 calories, no fat, and 1 gorgeous gram of fiber. So fill up a big bowl and munch to your heart's content—this is a great snack!

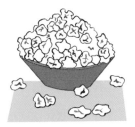

TABLE FOR ONE, PLEASE

Now that we've covered dining in, let's talk about eating out. A very important rite of passage in crossing the threshold back to singledom is to take yourself out on the town. Lunching at your favorite outdoor café can give you a great sense of strength, and can renew your commitment to treating yourself especially well during a difficult time.

When the menu arrives, don't be shy; order whatever you want, whether it's that bowl of pasta or that big piece of chocolate cake. This is the time to go all out! Take joy in pleasure wherever you can right now—you'll feel much better for the time being. Eventually your sources of happiness will be derived from other aspects of your life, but taking comfort in food can be a temporary poultice on a deep wound.

Splurge: Gooey Chocolate Brownies

Two Duncan Hines brownies have 320 calories and 14 grams of fat. Not terrible, but still more than a Snickers bar.

Solution: Vegan Chocolate Cake

This recipe takes no more than 10 minutes to make, and will keep your hands and mind occupied. You can make two large layers, or bake them in mini loaf pans and freeze one for future cravings.

3 CUPS FLOUR

2 CUPS SUGAR

6 TABLESPOONS COCOA

2 TEASPOONS BAKING SODA

1 TEASPOON SALT

¾ CUP VEGETABLE OIL

2 TABLESPOONS VINEGAR

2 TEASPOONS VANILLA

2 CUPS COLD WATER

Mix the dry ingredients together in a large bowl. Add the wet ingredients. Stir until smooth. Bake at 350 degrees F for 30 minutes. Makes two layers of a 9-inch round cake, or one cake baked in a loaf pan. When cool, make a lemon

glaze: combine 2 tablespoons confectioner's sugar with 2 teaspoons lemon juice. Whisk together until well combined and drizzle over cake.
Per one-inch slice, 275 calories and 9.6 grams of fat.

Splurge: Fluffernutter Sandwich on White Bread

Remember the peanut butter and fluff sandwich? It was the ultimate after-school snack. A fluffernutter sandwich has 390 calories and creates inner happiness, but it ain't got much in the nutritionally sound department—sorry to be the heavy here!

Solution: Almond Butter with All-Fruit Preserves on Whole-Grain Bread

Just a few small changes kicks the nutrient composition up a notch. Almond butter gives you more calcium than peanut butter (2 tablespoons of almond butter has 86 mg; peanut butter has none), as well as 3 grams of fiber and 1 ounce of protein. Both sandwiches have virtually the same amount of calories.

Splurge: General Tso's Chinese Chicken

General Tso's chicken is about the most dangerous Chinese dish on the menu—dark meat battered and deep-fried, then cooked with vegetables in a sweet (translation: sugary) and spicy sauce. A 2-cup serving size contains 830 calories, 37 grams of total fat, and 7 grams of saturated fat.

Solution: Szechuan Chicken

Szechuan chicken, made with lean white meat and sautéed vegetables, is a far better choice. Two cups contain 500 calories, 21 grams of total fat, and 2 grams of saturated fat. If you order steamed brown rice on the side, your fortune cookie will be sure to give you the blessing of health!

Splurge: French Fries

A medium serving of McDonald's French fries contains 350 calories and 18 grams of fat. Not the end of the world, but considering that they fry in cheap, unhealthful oils, there's a lot more danger to eating these than the numbers show. Plus, you're forgetting the Big Mac (560 calories) and the strawberry shake (740 calories) you'll probably order, which brings your meal total up to 1,650 calories.

REBOUND RITUALS

Listed below are some coping strategies to help you get through the initial shock and grief of a breakup.

Busy hands make happy hands: Let your creative juices flow by taking up a craft or repainting your walls.

Retail therapy: Shop till you drop.

Be your own storyteller: Record your tales of woe with new pens and a journal.

Kabuki war paint: Purchase new eye shadows and lipsticks.

Bedroom eyes: Try wearing false eyelashes for a little extra gla-*more*.

Put extra pep in your step: Treat your tootsies to a pedicure.

Be a bronze beauty: Counteract sallow post-breakup skin with self-tanning creams.

Say it with flowers: Treat yourself to a fresh bouquet.

New 'do, new you: Change your hairstyle.

Handle with care: Get a massage.

Choose your weapon of mass seduction: Wear your favorite undies!

Reach out and touch someone: Call your friends and family.

Watch sad movies.

Listen to your favorite albums.

Go dancing: Have a night out with the girls.

Soak it out: Draw yourself a luxurious bubble bath.

Solution: Baked Fries

Slice up a sweet potato, brush it with coconut oil and sprinkle on sea salt, and bake it on a cookie sheet in the oven for 45 minutes at 350 degrees F, or until crispy. Or you can buy frozen fries and simply reheat them in the oven; 200 calories per serving. That's what I'm talking about!

Splurge: Hot Chocolate

A tall Starbucks hot chocolate with whipped cream has 330 calories, 18 grams of fat, and 28 grams of sugar. Do yourself a favor and make your own, which costs much less and still satisfies your sweet craving.

Solution: Homemade Hot Chocolate

Heat 1 cup of skim milk or water just until it begins to boil. Remove from heat, and stir in 1 tablespoon unsweetened cocoa powder and 2 teaspoons of agave syrup. Add in some cinnamon and vanilla extract if you like, for extra punch, as well as a splash of whole milk. Agave syrup is derived from the nectar of the agave plant and is naturally low in sugar but high in flavor; it looks and tastes like honey. This has 130 calories if made with milk, 50 calories if made with water. If you like the taste of milk-based hot cocoa but are lactose-intolerant, try rice or almond milk, both of which make a delicious hot cocoa.

Splurge: Candy Bar

Standard-size chocolate bars (like Snickers, Hershey's milk chocolate, and Milky Way) supply roughly 250 calories, derived mostly from sugars and fat. Once in a blue moon it's an absolute treat, but don't make it a regular habit!

Solution: Dark Chocolate

Not only does dark chocolate satisfy your sweet tooth, but you'll get the benefits of antioxidants too! Plus, you may feel extra love when you eat chocolate. Phenylethylamine is a compound that naturally occurs in chocolate. When consumed, it releases endorphins in your brain that produce a mild feeling of euphoria, mimicking the sensation of being in love. Other compounds detected and measured in chocolate include serotonin, theobromine, and anandamide, which are all naturally occurring compounds that elevate mood, increase circulation, and enhance sensory perception. One ounce of dark chocolate (70 percent cocoa content or higher) contains about 154 calories, 12 grams of fat, 2 grams of fiber, and 2 grams of protein. Spread a little natural peanut butter on your chocolate if you'd like a homemade mini peanut butter cup!

Work It Out

After you've had your cake and eaten it too, you'll want to start getting back in shape again. Nothing gets your endorphins going more than a challenging stint on the treadmill. It's better to exhaust yourself working out than to exhaust yourself crying! And think of how good it will make you feel, because you'll get the natural antidepressant effects that exercise provides. What are the best exercises to do? Whatever ones you like. If you're a nature buff, head to the park for some tree-hugging and walk it out. Or strap on your Rollerblades and cruise at high velocity with the wind in your face. Or go for a few laps around the track, alternating slow jogging with fast sprints. Or hop on a bike and pedal it out. Whatever you do, remember that the goal is to clear your mind, and the side effect is fitness. What could be better? Don't forget other activities: swimming, jumping rope, yoga, Pilates, volleyball, basketball, golf, aerobics, spinning, and lifting weights. The gym is your oyster! If you feel unmotivated, try to get a friend to work out with you, or consider hiring yourself a personal trainer.

If you've been committed to working out for a while, then it's time to kick it up a notch and challenge yourself to participate in a competitive event. There is something so slick about donning a race number and a time chip. It changes your status from novice sideliner to plucky participant. Training for something you never thought you could do, and then completing it, will give you a huge rush and sense of accomplishment. Make your goals small

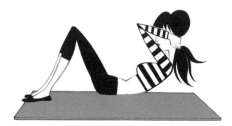

and attainable, like a three-mile walk or run, or a ten-mile bike ride. Keep it simple, so you know you can do it and do it well. Ask friends and family members to come cheer you on and take your picture, so you can be a rock star for a day. Talk about the ultimate morale booster!

Needle I Say More: Acupuncture

Getting stuck with needles may not sound like your idea of a good time, but this is an incredibly effective (and healthful) way to help you balance your chakras. Chakras are energy fields correlated with your nervous system and different organs in your body. Whether we are stressed, anxious, or just feeling off-kilter, a few guided needles, gently placed, can literally tap right into our nervous system and calm down a serious case of the jitters. Acupuncture is a fantastic adjunct to good nutrition, and can be used to treat many of the same ailments: hormonal imbalances, digestive issues, immune-function irregularities, and countless others. If working with a qualified practitioner is out of your price range, visit your local acupuncture school, where students will often work on you for heavily discounted rates.

The Rebirth of a New You

Breakups are the perfect time to reinvent yourself, journal what went wrong, and think about what you want to look for the next time around. Yes, you're going to be in a funk for a while, and you may feel sad, rejected, angry, and lonely. But over time, your process will become your journey, and when you've thought everything through and the anger is long gone, you'll be left with a tremendous sense of inner peace and knowing that there was a reason behind it all. Like a butterfly emerging from its cocoon, you are now ready to celebrate your newfound freedom, grab your girlfriends, and head out on the town!

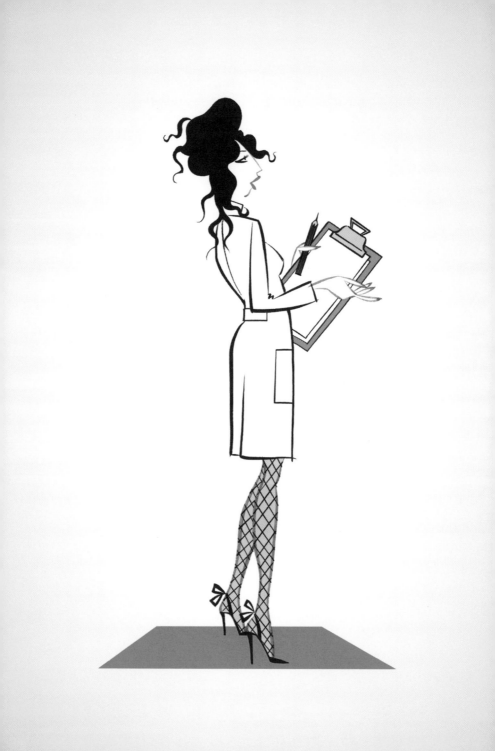

chapter 7

GORGEOUS
Questions and Answers

You can tell whether a man is clever by his answers.
You can tell whether a man is wise by his questions.—Naguib Mahfouz

FORGIVE ME, ESTHER, FOR I HAVE SINNED

So often, the brave souls who cross the threshold of my office mistake my
humble abode for a confessional booth. Not only do they fear having to con-
fess their every food sin, they fear that I'll demand some sort of repentance in
the form of a strict, Spartan diet for the months to come. Gorgeous, successful women crumble under the fear of what's to come by wolfing down jelly
doughnuts, Snickers bars, frozen yogurt, chocolate-covered pretzels, and
Cinnabons, because they think it's truly their Last Supper. Fear not, my little
food vixens, those of you who've read the previous chapters know that I'm
all about moderation—even moderation in moderation! Rather than feeling
victimized by your choices, it's possible to feel empowered by them—you just
need a few answers first. I've included here the questions I'm asked the most
often by clients, friends, and family. Hopefully you'll find some answers to
some of your more pressing questions too.

Q: Is it true that if I work out in the morning on an empty stomach I'll burn more calories? Or should I eat first?

A: All you early birds out there catching the worm, I applaud you! Research shows that exercising first thing in the morning on an empty stomach burns 30 percent more calories than exercising later on in the day! What's that sound? Do I hear angels singing?

However, there are two exceptions to this rule. The first exception is that if you are training for an endurance event and performing high-intensity exercise for more than an hour, you should definitely eat something before exercising; otherwise you'll deplete your glycogen stores. Glycogen is the fuel that powers your muscles. It is the stored form of carbohydrates that is retained in your liver and your muscles. Working out with inadequate glycogen stores will cause your performance to suffer, and the next day you'll be rewarded with sore, achy muscles laden with lactic acid. The second exception is that people with fast metabolisms may have a very hard time exercising on an empty stomach, and will need to eat beforehand. If this is the case for you, choose something energizing and easy to digest: Yogurt, fruit, and oatmeal are great choices.

What about you night-owl exercisers? Not to worry, you'll still reap fantastic benefits from your workout, but keep in mind that it will take your body at least thirty minutes to burn off stored glycogen before you start burning fat stores. Whether you exercise in the A.M. or the P.M., always exercise with a heart-rate monitor to minimize your output of stress hormones and help your body burn fat. Here's what I mean: During strenuous exercise, you can do your body more harm than good, because your adrenal glands will put out a stress hormone called cortisol, which breaks down muscle and stores your food as fat. Optimal fat burning occurs at a lower heart rate, when the body is in a highly oxygenated state. You can't start a fire burning (or, in your case, fat burning) without the presence of oxygen. But if your heart rate is too high, you'll burn sugar instead of fat. It's a fine line to walk, I know. To get an idea of where your heart rate should be to burn the most fat, subtract your age from 180 and use that number as the top of your upper-range heart rate during exercise. So if you're 30 years old, your heart rate should be between

140 and 150 beats per minute. Training in the right heart-rate zone ensures an efficient workout that will leave you energized rather than exhausted. Have fun!

Q: Is coffee bad for me? I'm addicted!

A: Ours is a totally overcaffeinated society. This is pretty unfortunate, because I have seen so many health and energy problems resolve themselves when people quit coffee. Now, to be fair, there are a few upsides to coffee. Coffee does contain antioxidants. Coffee has antidepressant properties. Coffee has been shown to improve cognitive function and performance. And among some health-care practitioners, it makes a hell of an enema. Ewww... But before you get too excited, it's important to understand that the downsides to coffee far outweigh the benefits.

- Coffee depletes your store of B vitamins, which metabolize and detoxify homocysteine. Homocysteine is an amino acid that can accumulate in your bloodstream and, ultimately, cause a heart attack. So make sure to supplement with B vitamins and folic acid if you are a coffee drinker—it can literally save your life.
- Coffee causes insomnia. Even one cup of coffee takes twenty-four hours to clear out of your system. Coffee causes ulcers and gastrointestinal distress. Between the acids in the coffee and all the sugar/sweetener/cream/coffee whitener, you've dumped a toxic overload in your system before you've even had breakfast!
- Coffee can worsen depression. Aside from the caffeine content, one of the reasons why it's so addicting is because it temporarily raises a neurotransmitter in our brain called dopamine—a feel-good chemical that our bodies naturally crave. After the coffee wears off, we experience a drop in dopamine that exacerbates depression. Fret not. It's not necessary to rely on coffee to get a lift in dopamine. To get that lift without the coffee, try taking the amino acid supplement phenylalanine, which is a precursor to L-tyrosine (see Chapter 5, "Vitamin G," for more information on this). This naturally occurring amino acid is readily available in most foods, particularly meats and milk products, with lower levels

found in oats and wheat germ. It is essential for many bodily functions and is one of the few amino acids that can cross the blood-brain barrier and therefore directly affect brain chemistry. Phenylalanine metabolism requires pyridoxine (P5P or vitamin B_6), niacin (vitamin B_3), vitamin C, copper, and iron. Phenylalanine is better absorbed than tyrosine and produces fewer headaches, so it may be more useful in treating depression than taking L-tyrosine directly.

- Coffee can make you tired and fat! Shocking, I know. But coffee increases the output of the stress hormone cortisol, which is produced in the adrenal glands. High cortisol levels result in a bigger waistline, insulin resistance, poor muscle tone, and a dip in energy levels between 3 and 4 P.M.
- What about decaf, you say? A wolf in sheep's clothing. Decaf contains more toxic chemicals than its regular, fully leaded counterparts, and still has 10 mg of caffeine per 8 ounces.

In a nutshell, I suggest weaning yourself off coffee. As outlined above, it does much more harm than good. You don't have to give up the hot beverages altogether. Switch to green tea, which is rich in antioxidants, helps your body oxidize fat, and won't give you the jittery effects of coffee.

Q: Can coffee give you heart palpitations?

A: Yes. Many of my patients have suffered from palpitations after drinking caffeinated coffee. Commercial varieties have up to 600 milligrams of caffeine per 12 ounces! Remember when we were kids and our parents only had a 6- or 8-ounce mug of coffee in the morning? Well, now the average American adult drinks 16 to 24 ounces of coffee per day—thanks in part to the coffee chains' huge cups. This much coffee puts *way* too much stress on the nervous system … no wonder we have so much road rage in this country! Coffee also depletes the body's supply of magnesium, which is a very calming trace mineral that normally relaxes the heart muscle.

Coffee isn't the only culprit causing heart palpitations. Exercise, smoking, alcohol, and stress are frequent causes of this problem. But most people find that cutting out coffee makes a big difference. If you cut out coffee and are still having palpitations, get your booty over to your doctor's office to get ruled out for mitral valve prolapse or a more serious underlying cause.

Q: Is it true that caffeine and alcohol dehydrate you? After a cup of coffee or a cocktail, I find I have to pee a lot more than usual, so it seems to me that it's hydrating me.

A: Caffeine and alcohol have an interesting effect on the system. Both naturally suppress ADH, or antidiuretic hormone. ADH's main job is to regulate the amount of water excreted by the kidneys. Too much caffeine and alcohol suppresses ADH, which causes the kidneys to flush water out of the system. Ultimately this lowers the fluid volume in your body, *et voilà*—dehydration ensues.

Q: I keep hearing that stress causes weight gain. How can this be true? You'd think that an elevated heart rate would burn more calories.

A: This question ties in nicely with the discussion above about coffee and cortisol levels; both stress and coffee raise cortisol levels, which can ultimately make you gain weight.

Cortisol is a necessary hormone that gives you the energy you need to begin your day. But as important and necessary as cortisol is, you can have too much of it circulating in your system. Under normal circumstances your body produces more cortisol in the morning than in the evening. In the evening your cortisol level should drop by approximately 90 percent. Evening is generally the time when the stresses of the day are behind you, the time when you can relax and unwind. But scientific data is showing that elevated cortisol levels are becoming more commonplace—especially in working women with children.

When we were kids, our cortisol levels could spike and then return to normal in a few hours. As adults, an hour or two of stress can take three to four days to resolve. Well, what if we're under stress all day long? Then we have chronically elevated cortisol levels, which can lead to health issues—one of them being weight gain. Research now correlates chronically elevated levels of cortisol with blood sugar problems, fat accumulation, compromised immune function, exhaustion, bone loss, and even heart disease. Memory loss has also been associated with high cortisol levels.

When the adrenals are not functioning properly and cortisol remains chronically elevated, the adrenal gland can wear itself out and no longer be able to produce even normal levels of cortisol. This is called adrenal exhaustion, and it renders the glands unable to meet your body's needs.

Lastly, new studies show that elevated cortisol levels can lead to an increase in abdominal fat, insulin resistance, and Type 2 diabetes.

How do you know if you have elevated cortisol? Unfortunately, it's not something you can immediately feel. If it is elevated for too long a period—for months or even years, for example—you may feel wired but tired and burned out most of the time. If you suspect you're at risk, a blood, urine, or saliva hormone test for cortisol can be an excellent red flag that it's time for you to be proactive and take stress-reducing measures. Even if you don't think you're at high risk for high cortisol levels, it's not a bad idea to check them before they get too high. The good news is that anyone can lower or maintain their cortisol levels with stress management and supplements. Even ten minutes of yoga per day can help lower your levels! So don't give up—keep the faith, sister. Please also see Chapter 5, "Vitamin G," for supplement protocols for reducing your cortisol levels.

Q: Which are better for you, peanut M&M's or plain ones?

A: From both a personal and a professional perspective, I'd choose peanut M&M's any day! The peanuts contain protein and essential fatty acids that will slow down the release of the sugar into the bloodstream. I just ask that you buy yourself a small bag rather than the two-pounder; no amount of peanuts will save your blood sugar at that point!

Q: Is diet soda really bad for me? I love it!

A: In a word: YES! Now, you're talking to a girl who loves Diet Coke with lemon, but the stuff is pretty toxic. Diet sodas are loaded with aspartame and/or other artificial sweeteners that compete with serotonin-uptake receptors on the brain. Because these chemicals work in a "lock and key" method, this disrupts normal nerve cell communication by preventing neurotransmitters from sending information from neuron to neuron. Yikes! If you struggle with depression, insomnia, bulimia, obsessive-compulsive behavior, or general moodiness, diet soda will just exacerbate the problem. And that's not even the worst of it: There are at least ninety-two different health side effects associated with aspartame consumption, including brain tumors, birth defects, diabetes, emotional disorders, epilepsy, and seizures. Further, when aspartame is stored for long periods of time or kept at warm temperatures, it changes to methanol, an alcohol that converts to formaldehyde and formic acid, which are known carcinogens and deadly neurotoxins. An EPA assessment of methanol states that it "is considered a cumulative poison due to the low rate of excretion once it is absorbed." The EPA recommends a limit of consumption of 7.8 mg per day. A one-liter (approximately one-quart) aspartame-sweetened beverage contains about 56 mg of methanol. If aspartame-sweetened soda is stored in a warm place, the health risks increase further.

Aside from the negative effects of the ingredients, drinking a lot of soda is likely to leave you with little appetite for vegetables, protein, and other food that your body needs. All soda, be it diet or regular, is unhealthy for you. Try body-friendly versions of flavored seltzers or unflavored seltzer with lemons and limes to wean yourself off the liquid crack you've been chugging.

Q: I keep hearing that fish is good for you. But at the same time, I hear that farm-grown salmon is bad, and other fish have mercury. What are the safest fishes to eat? I also don't want to spend twenty dollars a pound on fish.

A: Look, I hate to be Debbie Downer here, but we need to get the message out that methylmercury, a poisonous substance, is in most of the fish we eat. How did methylmercury make its way into fish? It's a sad story: Each year, thousands of tons of mercury are released into the air through pollution and waste. In the environment this mercury turns into organic mercury, which is known as methylmercury, and accumulates in streams, oceans, water, and soil.

Methylmercury then makes its way into the food chain. A little fish eats some contaminated plankton, a bigger fish eats several little fish, thereby absorbing more methylmercury, and an even bigger fish eats several of those fish, and so on. For this reason, larger and older fish, such as sharks and swordfishes, contain the highest levels of methylmercury. And people who regularly eat fish have higher levels of methylmercury than those who don't. Pregnant or breastfeeding women who eat a lot of fish put their newborns at risk, as methylmercury can harm a developing baby's brain and nervous system. Other groups that are particularly sensitive to mercury exposure include children under the age of six years, people with impaired kidney function, and people with sensitive immune responses to metals. I've seen it in my practice and have experienced mercury toxicity firsthand. Avoid toxic fishes if you can—it's no picnic to be sick! If you experience memory loss, weight gain, low thyroid function, diarrhea, headaches and/or "brain fog," irregular heartbeat, or insomnia, or you have a mouth full of silver fillings, get yourself to a holistic M.D. and get yourself checked out for mercury toxicity.

What about farm-raised fishes, you ask? Steer clear, my friend! Farm-raised fish do not eat the same wholesome diet as wild fish. Instead they are fed grains like corn, and these grains do not form the beneficial omega-3 fatty acids. Without these fatty acids, you will not receive all the benefits that many studies ascribe to eating fish. Farm-raised fish may also be exposed to tremendously high pesticide levels from runoff from nearby agricultural crops, which are usually heavily sprayed.

So which fish are the safest to eat? Those that are wild and/or low in mercury. Your best bet is wild Alaskan salmon. Farm-raising fish is illegal in Alaska, so the gorgeous creatures are allowed to swim and spawn in their natural habitat and grow in clean waters. The other upside to eating wild Alaskan salmon is that they are rich in the essential omega-3 fatty acids, free of PCBs, rich in DMAE (which contributes to cognitive function and muscle tone), and leaner than their farm-raised counterparts, which have a much higher concentration of saturated fat. Yes, I do agree that it is more expensive to eat wild fish instead of farmed, but as someone who has now gone through two detoxes trying to pull the mercury out of my body, I am willing to pay the price rather than deal with problems from mercury toxicity down the road. Beware of wild salmon sold in grocery stores, however. Though mislabeling food is against the law, multiple exposés in the *New York Times* have verified cases of vendors across the country selling farm-raised salmon as wild. Federal regulations have begun requiring that fish carry a paper trail back to their source, but these rules apply only to full-service markets such as grocery stores, and not to fish markets. Visit www.VitalChoice.com for a clean and reputable source of mercury-free fish from Alaska.

Other great sources of low-mercury fish include sardines, herring, halibut, catfish (farmed), blue crab (mid-Atlantic), croaker, flounder (summer), haddock, trout (farmed), and shrimp.

What are PCBs? PCBs are a group of toxic, carcinogenic organic compounds that were used until 1979 in the manufacture of plastics and as insulating fluids in electrical transformers and capacitors. They behave much like DDT in the environment in that they are very stable compounds and are also fat-soluble; therefore, they accumulate in ever-higher concentrations as they move up the food chain. The use of PCBs was banned in the United States, but they still exist in the environment.

Q: I'm in my thirties and my face looks like it is experiencing the hormones of my teenage years. What can I change in my diet that will help?

A: Oy. So many factors, so little time. I can tell you that if you really and truly are dedicated to the cause, you can clear up your skin. I know this because it has worked not only on me but on my patients. However, you *must* commit to the program. First and foremost, cut out all wheat and dairy, except yogurt, for one month. Secondly, take six omega-3 fatty acid capsules per day. Third, take probiotic (e.g., acidophilus or bifidobacteria) capsules or powder with food at a dose of 8 to 16 billion organisms per day. Fourth, ditch the coffee and switch to green or black tea. Last, do not even think of sugar or beer or any other yeast-containing foods. You'll be looking gorgeous again in just a matter of weeks.

Q: I feel like I can never get enough sleep. Is it my diet?

A: It might be. Your first task is to be wary of grains and sugars. These temporarily raise your blood sugar and inhibit sleep. Later, when your blood sugar drops too low (hypoglycemia), you're likely to wake up and not be able to fall back asleep. So try to skip the chocolate bar or the ice cream before bed. The same goes for alcohol, one of the worst sleep disruptors of all. Hey, don't shoot the messenger, babes! I'm just telling you what I know. Also check in with yourself about that morning caffeine habit of yours. As I said earlier, the caffeine in a cup of coffee takes a full 24 hours to leave the system.

To help you sleep through the night, eat a high-protein snack a few hours before bed. This will provide the L-tryptophan your body needs to produce melatonin and serotonin—your brain's built-in sleep aids. It also helps if you eat a small piece of fruit with your protein to help the tryptophan cross the blood-brain barrier.

While diet plays a big role in the quality of sleep, there are other things you can do to help you get through the night. Following are some suggestions for a good night's rest:

- **Sleep in a darkened room.** Even the tiniest bit of light in the room can disrupt your circadian rhythms and your pineal gland's production of melatonin and serotonin. Use an eye mask to keep out any light coming through the window. Also try to keep the light off if you get up during the night. As soon as you turn on that light you will immediately cease all production of the important sleep aid melatonin for the rest of the night.

- **Breathe before bed to lower your cortisol.** People with chronic insomnia have increased blood levels of stress hormones and suffer from sustained, round-the-clock activation of the body's system for responding to stress. Ten minutes of yoga, stretching, or meditative breathing will lower your cortisol levels before bed.

- **Exercise regularly.** Exercising for at least thirty minutes every day can help you fall asleep. But try not to exercise too close to bedtime or it may keep you awake. Studies show that exercising in the morning, if you can do it, is the best for insomnia.

- **Journaling.** If you often lie in bed with your mind racing, it might be helpful to keep a journal on your nightstand and write down your thoughts before bed.

- **Try to get to bed before 11 P.M.** Our adrenal glands do most of their recovering during the hours from 11 P.M. to 1 A.M. If you can't go to bed early, at least be consistent about the time you go to bed and the time you wake up.

- **Take a hot bath or shower before bed.** Raising your body temperature in the late evening will ensure that it falls at bedtime, facilitating sleep.

- **Keep the clock out of sight.** Looking at the time and thinking about the sleep you're missing will only add to your worry. Try to ignore the clock during the middle of the night so you can fall back asleep without stressing about the time.

- **Use your bed only for sleeping and sex.** If you are used to watching TV or doing work in bed, you may find it harder to relax and to think of the bed as a place to sleep.

- **Have sex, either with your partner or yourself.** What, you thought I wouldn't mention it? Oh, come *on.* Enough said.

Q: My busy schedule makes it hard for me to eat regular meals. Can you recommend a good, healthful snack to take the edge off so that I don't binge on the candy or other junk foods taunting me in our office kitchen?

A: Oh, I can recommend many, my dear! Why stop at one? Let's see . . . a handful of raw nuts and seeds, celery with natural peanut butter, a hard-boiled egg, plain yogurt sweetened with fruit and honey, turkey slices rolled up with guacamole inside them, and fresh fruit will all make your taste buds tingle and keep your energy fired up throughout the day. Try to snack at least twice a day to keep your metabolic fires stoked, and to promote fat burning. This means that if you eat breakfast at 8 A.M., you should have a snack between 10 and 11 A.M., lunch at 1 P.M., another snack at 4 P.M., and dinner by 8 P.M.

Q: Is it okay to take all of my vitamins at once (as opposed to two divided doses) each day? Where should I go to get the best form of vitamins? How do I figure out which vitamins make sense for my body makeup?

A: In a perfect world, we would all take our vitamins in two or three divided doses throughout the day. But reality usually dictates that we slam down a fistful of pills with our breakfast before madly dashing out the door to work. Just do your best, darling, and remember this: Vitamins are always better in your body than in the bottle!

To get the best form of vitamins and determine which ones you should take, work with a holistic nutritionist or nutritionally oriented physician. I can tell you that in my practice I recommend a combination of food-based and commercially made vitamins, depending on the needs of the individual. Yes, you can get by with supplements from the Vitamin Shoppes or GNCs of the world, but it's better to consult a health-care practitioner who can focus on your personal needs. When you seek the guidance of a professional practitioner, you are paying for the practitioner's time spent researching and figuring out what will be best for you. So for the best quality of pills coupled with the best advice, look no further than your local healers, who offer a wealth of knowledge!

Q: Which vitamins are helpful when I can't get enough sleep?

A: It really is a shame when a girl just can't get her beauty rest. It wreaks havoc on your mood, slows your motor coordination, decreases your cognitive function, and makes your skin look tired, to boot. We've all been there, haven't we? Rather than rely on caffeine and sugar to pep you up, try energizing your body with nutrients, which can be just as effective, and for longer periods of time. To put some pep in your step, try the following cocktail with your breakfast:

> *1,000 mg of L-carnitine*
>
> *300 mg of lipoic acid*
>
> *50 mg of B-complex vitamins*
>
> *1 teaspoon of licorice root in tincture form*
>
> *1 teaspoon of ashwagandha root in tincture form*

If you're really ambitious, you can take these with a shot of wheatgrass, which also contains hundreds of vitamins and trace minerals. Together, these nutrients fuel your cells' mitochondria, or powerhouses, which are responsible for energy production. These nutrients will also support the adrenal glands, which stabilize your blood sugar and regulate your output of stress hormones.

Q: What do you think about eggs—are they friend or foe?

A: Egg-cellent question, *ma petite cherie*. Eggs have been given a bad rap, and for no good reason. Clear room on the soapbox here and pay attention, everybody: *Eggs never have raised and never will raise your cholesterol.* And if that doesn't blow your mind, consider the fact that the yolks have more protein than the whites and contain the brain-protective nutrients lecithin and choline. Buy the organic kind enriched with EPA/DHA for a delicious and healthful product.

Q: Does eating at night make you fatter?

A: This is probably the one question I get asked most often. If you are going to eat right before bed, make it a very small portion. Otherwise you'll spend your sleep time digesting, which can disrupt your sleep cycle. I don't think you have to stop eating past a certain cutoff time, but be mindful of the types of foods you are consuming and make them healthful ones.

Q: Why does my pee smell funny and turn green after I eat asparagus?

A: Asparagus is packed with amino acids that break down during digestion into six sulfur-containing compounds. These compounds are responsible for the odor. Although it's stinky and can make interesting dinner party conversation, it's a harmless and temporary effect.

One school of thought says that about half of all people have a gene enabling us to break down the sulfurous amino acids in asparagus into their smellier components. Others think that everyone digests asparagus the same way, but only about half of us have a gene that enables us to smell the specific compounds formed in the digestion of asparagus.

Q: Is it really healthy to drink one glass of red wine a day?

A: That, my friend, is the $64,000 question. No definitive answer exists, so I'll answer like a scientist: It depends. Drinking one glass of red wine each day appears to be beneficial in preventing heart disease and may extend your lifespan. Red wine is rich in the antioxidant resveratrol, and resveratrol belongs to a family of compounds known as polyphenols. Polyphenols are known to combat damaging free radicals in the body. Resveratrol also lowers "bad" LDL cholesterol while raising "good" HDL cholesterol and decreases the production of a protein that plays a major role in the development of heart disease. But proceed with caution, my little tippler: two or more glasses a day can impair liver function and undo all the good benefits of that one glass a day. And if you have a history of diabetes, high blood pressure, or yeast infections, proceed with caution.

Q: Why do bananas make me feel tired?

A: Two potential reasons: One is that you're allergic to them, and the other is that the high sugar and starch content soaks into your bloodstream at a rapid pace, temporarily raising your blood sugar. About an hour later, you'll crash and burn and your energy levels will poop out. The moral of the story? Eat bananas with some peanut butter or another source of protein to blunt the entry of sugar into the bloodstream.

Q: I'm confused by all the info on organic foods. What does the "organic" label really mean? Is organic produce nutritionally superior to nonorganic produce?

A: Technically speaking, certified organic food must be free from all genetically modified organisms, be produced without artificial pesticides or fertilizers, and (for meat) be from an animal raised without the routine use of antibiotics, growth promoters, or other drugs. However, many food producers interpret these rules differently, so for the most current information, visit www.organicconsumers.org.

Research shows that organic produce is indeed superior to nonorganic produce. Aside from pesticide contamination, conventional produce tends to have fewer nutrients than organic produce; on average, conventional produce has only 83 percent of the nutrients of organic produce. Studies have found significantly higher levels of nutrients such as vitamin C, iron, magnesium, and phosphorus, and significantly less nitrates (a toxin) in organic crops. But bear in mind that nonorganic veggies are better than no veggies, so try not to make yourself crazy about eating only organic. For when I can't find good organic produce, I keep on hand a pesticide wash (try your local health-food store) that removes some of the chemical residues from the vegetables.

Q: If you could afford to eat only one food group organically, which would it be? Meat, dairy, fruits and veggies?

A: If I had to pick, I'd definitely choose to eat meat and dairy from grass-fed animals. Grass-fed meats are free of the hormones and antibiotics present in commercially raised meats and poultry. These hormones and antibiotics can disrupt our endocrine and immune systems. Bear in mind, however, that organically raised animals may still be fed corn or soy, which can make the meat higher in saturated fat, because it is still not what nature intended them to eat. At the top of the list are organically raised grass-fed animals and the meats and the milk they produce; their meat has more omega-3s than fish! Grass-fed meats are naturally low in fat and also less likely to be tainted with mad cow disease. You can find these meats and dairy products in organic food markets or online.

Q: Why does iceberg lettuce get such a bad rap?

A: Ever hear the expression "the darker the berry, the sweeter the juice"? Well, the same goes for fruits and veggies—the deeper the color, the greater the nutritional value. If you feel you just can't cross over from iceberg to spinach, try Bibb or Boston lettuce for a happy medium.

Q: As an athletic person, how do I know if I'm getting enough protein?

A: Some experts would say that it depends on the type of exercise you do. Some think that weight lifters should cram in protein like there's no tomorrow, while long-distance runners should load up on pasta. But guess what? Both groups need to make sure they get adequate protein. Contrary to popular belief, cardiovascular workouts require as much protein as weight lifting. To determine your daily protein needs, divide your body weight by 2.2

to determine your weight in kilograms. If you are sedentary and are sitting on your booty all day, multiply your kilogram weight by 1.0–1.2 grams per kilogram. If you work out one to three times per week and work up a good sweat, multiply your weight by 1.2–1.5 grams per kilogram. If you work out three to five times per week, multiply your weight by 1.5–1.7 grams per kilogram. And if you're working out six or seven days per week, you sicko, then you will need a whopping 2.0 grams per kilogram of protein. Good luck!

Q: What are the best pre-and post-workout snacks?

A: Anything you eat within an hour of working out should be easy to digest: Fresh fruit, diluted pomegranate juice, or a cup of plain low-fat yogurt with honey are simple carbohydrates that will be absorbed quickly into the bloodstream to fuel your muscles during your workouts. Within one hour of finishing your workout, eat a combination of protein, fat, and carbohydrates to refuel your glycogen stores; try oatmeal with sliced almonds and berries, half a turkey sandwich with avocado and tomato slices, or chicken with sautéed spinach and lentils.

Q: I've been feeling lethargic during my workouts and think it may be related to my nutrition. Any thoughts?

A: First and foremost, make sure you're getting enough sleep. Second, keep a food log and take inventory of what you're eating. Then try this: For one month, eliminate all processed foods (white flour, pasta, white rice, white sugar, pizza, crackers, muffins, and breads). Stick to whole foods, such as lean proteins, fresh fruits and veggies, avocados, nuts and seeds, lentils and beans, barley, and steel-cut oats. Then add back your favorite foods one at a time, every fourth day, and record in your food log how you feel. I guarantee that the foods you are (or aren't) eating are causing your energy problems.

Q: What about protein powders and protein bars? Are these good substitutes when you're on the run?

A: Protein bars can be a relatively healthy snack if need be, but don't go too crazy eating them. They're not meant to replace meals. Instead, use them as a backup plan when you can't find anything else healthful nearby, when you're on a hike, or when you're traveling and want to avoid skanky airplane food. I recommend bars that are (surprise, surprise) made from whole foods. Steer clear of artificially sweetened bars with a lot of freaky chemical-laden ingredients. Look for ingredients like almond butter, agave syrup, date paste, and whey protein. Whey protein is the best protein powder on the market. It's a complete protein and can boost the immune system. Although whey protein is derived from dairy, it is virtually lactose-free, and most people seem to tolerate it just fine.

A great way to incorporate whey is in a homemade smoothie. Try this recipe by yours truly:

1 SCOOP WHEY PROTEIN (SHOULD CONTAIN 20 TO 30 GRAMS OF
    PROTEIN PER SCOOP)
1 CUP FROZEN BERRIES OR 1 BANANA
1 TABLESPOON NATURAL PEANUT OR ALMOND BUTTER
2 TABLESPOONS GROUND FLAXSEEDS
1 CUP WATER

Combine all ingredients in a blender with ice and a dash of cinnamon and blend well.

Q: I don't eat red meat and worry that I don't get enough iron. What are the best sources of iron, and how much do I need?

A: Meat-free sources of iron include oysters, poultry, salmon, beans, whole grains, eggs (especially egg yolks), and dried fruits. Mixing these foods with vitamin C–rich foods such as tomatoes, strawberries, green bell peppers, citrus fruits, broccoli, turnip greens and other leafy greens, sweet potatoes, and cantaloupe can improve your absorption of vegetable sources of iron up to three times!

Don't bother eating iron-fortified cereal, because the calcium in the milk you add to your cereal will inhibit the absorption of iron. Also bear in mind that iron from vegetables, fruits, grains, and supplements is harder for the body to absorb than iron from meat and fish.

If you take a supplement, 18 mg per day will do the trick. Do not take your iron with calcium supplements, dairy products, zinc, or tea; these will all inhibit iron absorption.

Q: Should I eat more red meat during my period?

A: It makes perfect sense to eat more red meat and liver during your period, especially if your periods are heavy. You may even find you crave meat around the time of your period, which is completely normal. Since you are losing blood and iron, your body will need to make up for these losses by getting extra dietary iron.

Q: Is it possible to take too much calcium?

A: Yes, it is possible to take too much calcium, especially if you have a history of kidney stones. However, for anyone without a history of kidney stones, there is no increased risk of developing kidney stones if you increase your calcium intake. Teenagers require 1,300 mg of calcium per day, adults 18 to 50 years old require 1,000 mg per day, and adults over 50 years require 1,200 mg per day.

To optimize your bone health, remember that it takes a village of nutrients to build bones. Calcium alone won't do it; 1,000 IU of vitamin D is essential to regulate the intestinal efficiency of calcium, and 400 to 800 mg per day of magnesium is important for parathyroid function, which also regulates calcium absorption and utilization in the body. Without adequate vitamin D, the intestine absorbs only 10 to 15 percent of dietary calcium; with adequate vitamin D, the intestine absorbs 30 to 80 percent! So the recommendation for calcium requirements should be based on the fact that sufficient vitamin D is present.

For you lucky gals who live in sunny climates, fifteen minutes of sunscreen-free sun exposure three times per week will also enable your body to make the vitamin D it needs through the skin. And if you're thinking that you eat plenty of dairy products and so you don't need to take vitamin D, think again: ice cream, yogurt, and cheese do *not* contain vitamin D. According to Michael Holick, the world's vitamin D expert, 21 percent of skim milk tested nationwide had undetectable levels of vitamin D! Shiver me timbers!

Q: On those nights when I can't get it together to actually make something, what kind of prepared foods (i.e. frozen dinners) are actually good for me?

A: There aren't a lot of quality prepared meals on the market. The truth hurts, my darling, and here's something else that will pain you: Just because it's organic doesn't mean it's good for you.

In the name of good research, this sexy scientist dove headfirst into the organic frozen foods section. I sniffed around, I scanned the labels, I turned over the products, and I furiously scribbled down notes (this is what us Virgos do). So here's the skinny: Most of them are overly processed and loaded with carbs, cheese, and tofu and really don't offer enough protein or nutritional balance. The good news is that they can be a healthy choice as long as you supplement the frozen meal with fresh side dishes. So you can have your chicken breast, spinach, and frozen entrée of pesto tortellini and eat it too. For instance, if you're going to eat a frozen chicken entrée, make sure you enjoy it with a side of steamed veggies and a salad, to boost the antioxidant component of the meal. Or if your frozen meal consists of pasta, then beef it up with ground turkey in tomato sauce and sautéed spinach with garlic.

Q: Can you suggest ways to order in a healthy dinner that will also provide leftovers for a healthy lunch? And what should I definitely avoid?

A: Although ordering takeout seems so easy ("I'll have the chicken enchilada with extra cheese, a side of refried beans, and tortilla chips with guacamole and salsa"), we do relinquish a lot of control when we turn over our meal prep to the voice at the other end of the phone. Will it be hot when you get it? Will it taste as good as when you have it in the restaurant? How much will you really get? Try this: The next time you order out, divide the portion in half and put one half away for tomorrow's lunch. If what you eat fills you up, you'll know you've had enough. As for healthy choices, you should place stock in how the food is prepared. Try to steer clear of fried or heavy foods, such as French fries, crackling or sizzling foods, heavy sauces, and creamed foods. Steaming, sautéing, and grilling are much better options. My favorite thing to do is to order sides of steamed veggies, then dress them up with olive oil, lemon, and garlic. Sashimi and miso soup are healthy order-in items, though you must eat them within forty-eight hours for food-safety reasons. International options work well too: tandoori chicken with yogurt sauce and chana saag; steamed chicken with lentils and veggies, brown sauce on the side; and a whole wheat burrito with black beans, chicken, peppers, and onions topped with guacamole and salsa all rank high on the Gorgeous Girl meal scale!

Well, there you have it, folks—real questions from real people just like you and me. Hopefully I've shed some light on the questions that've been lurking in your minds for days, months, years even! I hope you never stop seeking answers, because nutrition affects the quality of your life every day. Ta ta for now.

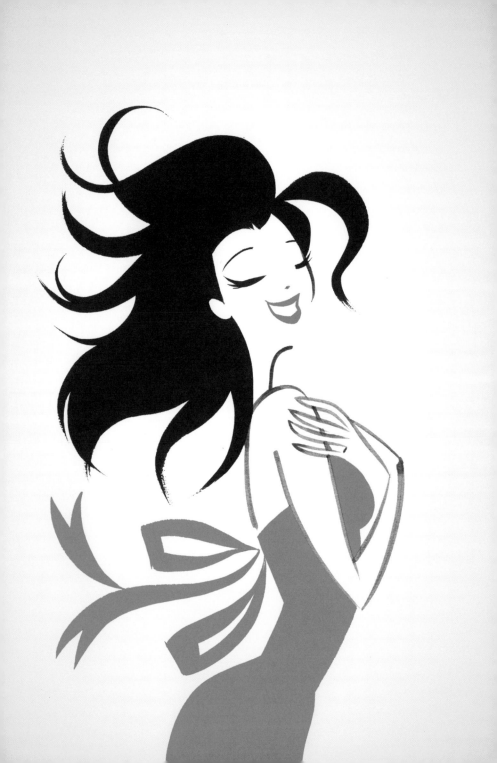

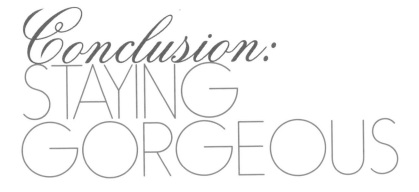

Conclusion: STAYING GORGEOUS

Later that day I got to thinking about relationships. There are those that open you up to something new and exotic, those that are old and familiar, those that bring up lots of questions, those that bring you somewhere unexpected, those that bring you far from where you started, and those that bring you back. But the most exciting, challenging and significant relationship of all is the one you have with yourself. And if you find someone to love the you you love, well, that's just fabulous. —Carrie Bradshaw, *Sex and the City*

You are now the mistress of my best-kept secrets. I hope you've come away with a glitter-encrusted, personally designed tool belt loaded with goodies to help you through thick and thin. Sure, there will be times when you push your body to the limit and party just a little too hard. That's okay as long as you remember that being a Gorgeous Girl means striking a balance between having fun and taking care of yourself. It means treating yourself as well as you'd treat a prized pair of Jimmy Choos—with respect and care. And last but not least, it means letting your hair down and having fun! Before I send you on your gorgeous way, there are a few more nuggets of wisdom I'd like to impart.

DOTE YOUR I'S

As women, we tend to spend most of our energy on the people we love and on our careers, but we don't always pay ourselves the fabulous attention we deserve. It's essential to make time to dote on yourself. This means not only splurging on the occasional mani-pedi, but also thinking about what motivates you to eat and live well. Enjoy your magnificent body, pamper your insides and outs, and revel in every single delicious indulgence and positive choice. There is no escaping the fact that we must be present in our own body at all times; our spirit is also always with us. So it behooves us to make peace with our bodies and our spirits. We need to recognize what we love about ourselves, what we'd like to improve upon, and what makes us special and unique. Maybe you know how to make the perfect batch of brownies. Maybe you're a fantastic listener, and friends come to you when they need the heal-ing properties of a soul mate. Maybe you write beautiful poems and give them to your loved ones as special pieces from the heart. Maybe you throw fabulous cocktail parties and know how to mix the perfect combination of friends. Whatever your special talent is, hold on to it and celebrate it. Over time, our bodies all change. There's not a darn thing we can do about it. So it's no use obsessing. Instead, focus on what makes you *you*. That's what will sustain you, no matter what your dress size or how you're eating that day.

TOO LEGIT TO QUIT

We can't ignore the fact that our eating is a direct reflection of what's going on in our lives: We eat the way we live and live the way we eat. As you and your life change, your eating habits will mirror those shifts. And sometimes taking a moment and looking at what you are eating helps you delve deeper into what's eating you. If you find yourself heading down an unhealthy road, it is usually temporary, and you'll get through it by paying more attention to the lessons you learned from this book. If you can't seem to shake the health blues, it might be because you need a healthy dose of attention to yourself. Paying attention to your health might be the first tangible step to recognizing and addressing other issues in your life. When you feel stressed about your eating or your life veering off-track, come back to this book. It will help.

So many times, we reach our target goal (such as achieving a certain weight or meeting the man of our dreams) and think that our journey is over—that we can sit back and rest on our laurels for a while. But the real journey entails enjoying what you have and who you are, whether you are up or down, trying to attain a goal or basking in your achievements. Just as many times you don't fit into your skinny jeans, you are going to have nights when you turn every head. Sometimes you will crave a tall glass of cold, cold water, and sometimes you will feel the need to throw back a beer. Either way, maintaining balance will keep you happy and healthy in the long run.

As a Gorgeous Girl, you know how to get to the good and handle the bad. And *that* is living well.

EAT, DRINK, AND BE GORGEOUS

I hope this book has inspired you to do some remodeling from within. And I hope I have been able to show you that being healthy can be fun—it's not just about flaxseeds and yoga. True, healthful food and supplements can have a dramatic effect on your body, mind, and spirit. But eating, drinking, and being gorgeous is 100 percent about living well and 100 percent about living it up.

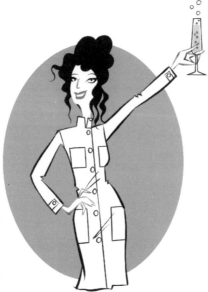

GLOSSARY OF GORGEOUS SUPPLEMENTS

Aqueous Selenium: Selenium is an essential trace mineral that has powerful antioxidant effects in the body. Selenium is also necessary for efficient energy production in the cell's furnace, the mitochondria, and for optimal functioning of the immune system. Aqueous selenium is particularly useful in treating mercury toxicity.

Ashwagandha Root: Used in Ayurvedic medicine, and sometimes called "Indian ginseng," this herb is native to India and Africa. Ashwagandha contains compounds called withanolides, which are similar to the active constituents in ginseng. Ashwagandha helps the body adapt better to environmental stresses, enhances immune function, and promotes an overall feeling of well-being.

Astragalus Root: Astragalus is a Chinese herb used to boost the immune system and reduce the adverse effects of stress and fatigue. It helps raise the white blood cell count and fight chronic viruses but should not be used if you have an acute infection or a fever.

Betaine Hydrochloride: Betaine hydrochloride is an acidic form of betaine, a vitamin-like substance found in grains and other foods. Betaine hydrochloride is recommended by some doctors as a supplemental source of hydrochloric acid for people who have a deficiency of stomach acid (hypochlorhydria). Gastric acid is produced by the parietal cells of the stomach to ward off bacterial and parasitic intestinal infections and to digest protein properly. If you are passing a lot of stinky gas, this is for you!

Borage Oil or GLA (Gamma Linoleic Acid): GLA is the active ingredient found in the oil of borage seeds. It is an essential fatty acid in the

Omega-6 category, but unlike the unhealthful Omega-6 oils, such as vegetable oil, borage oil has tremendous health-promoting effects. It is essential for smooth, healthy skin and helps women with hormonal balance, easing conditions such as PMS and menopause. GLA has been researched for its ability to relieve PMS, reduce inflammation caused by arthritis, lower cholesterol, and help reverse diabetic neuropathy.

Boswellia: Boswellia is an herb with anti-inflammatory benefits. It helps relieve joint pain, Crohn's disease, ulcerative colitis, and asthma. Boswellia also helps detoxify the joints, which often act as reservoirs for environmental toxins and stress.

Calcium Lactate: There is more calcium in the human body than all of the other minerals combined. Your body needs it every day, not just to keep your bones and teeth strong over your lifetime, but to ensure the proper functioning of your muscles and nerves. It even helps your blood clot. Calcium lactate is a very absorbable form of calcium.

Chaste Tree: Chaste tree promotes a natural, healthy balance within the female endocrine system, supports female reproductive health, and eases temporary feelings of tension associated with the menstrual cycle. Chaste tree berries normalize irregular menstrual periods and relieve PMS symptoms such as bloating, breast tenderness, and moodiness. *Note:* Do *not* take chaste tree if you are on the pill.

Chromium Picolinate: Chromium is an essential trace mineral that is vital for blood sugar regulation and energy production. It's important in processing carbohydrates and fats, and it helps cells respond properly to insulin—the hormone produced in the pancreas that makes blood sugar available to the cells as our basic fuel. It is therefore a key nutrient for people with diabetes, high triglycerides, and insulin resistance.

DIM (Diindolylmethane): DIM, a naturally occurring phytonutrient found in cruciferous vegetables, works by increasing the body's production of the beneficial forms of estrogen, while decreasing the two forms of bad estrogen that are linked to tumor growth. DIM is an excellent therapy for treating uterine fibroid tumors, fibrocystic breasts, and the symptoms of hormonal imbalance.

DMAE (Dimethylaminoethanol): A compound found in high levels in anchovies and sardines, DMAE enhances cognitive function; small amounts of it are also naturally produced in the human brain. It increases levels of the neurotransmitter acetylcholine in the brain, making it beneficial for improving short-term memory and concentration.

D-Mannose: Studies suggest that D-mannose is ten times more effective than cranberries in dislodging E. coli bacteria from the bladder wall and can ameliorate more than 90 percent of UTIs in twenty-four to forty-eight hours.

D-mannose is a naturally occurring sugar similar in structure to, but metabolized differently from, glucose (a component of table sugar). Because the body metabolizes only small amounts of D-mannose and excretes the rest in the urine, it doesn't interfere with blood sugar regulation, even in diabetics.

The cell wall of the UTI-causing E. coli bacteria has tiny fingerlike projections that contain complex molecules called lectins on their surfaces. These lectins act as a cellular glue that binds the bacteria to the bladder wall, so that they cannot be readily rinsed out by urination. However, because D-mannose molecules will glom on to these lectins and fill up all of the bacterial anchoring sites, the bacteria can no longer attach to the bladder wall and are, therefore, flushed away. In other words, unlike antibiotics, D-mannose does not kill any bacteria, whether they are good or bad, but simply helps displace them. Use the powdered form for optimal dosing.

Echinacea: An herb that works to both prevent and treat allergies, colds, and flus; support a weakened or suppressed immune system; and help with post-viral syndromes. Contrary to popular belief, it is safe for long-term use. Gargling with liquid echinacea can resolve a sore throat or swollen glands within twenty-four hours if used at the first signs of the symptoms. It should make your tongue feel numb, which lets you know you're using a product with active ingredients. Good luck; it will also make you cough and sputter as if you've taken a straight shot of whiskey!

Evening Primrose Oil: Evening primrose oil is derived from the seeds of the evening primrose plant. Like borage oil, EPO contains gamma linoleic acid (GLA) and can help relieve the symptoms of PMS, diabetes, and such inflammatory conditions as ulcerative colitis, lupus, and rheumatoid arthritis.

5-HTP (5-Hydroxytryptophan): 5-HTP is an amino acid that is the intermediate step between tryptophan and the important brain chemical serotonin. In this stress-filled era, the lifestyle and dietary practices of many people can cause lower levels of serotonin within the brain. As a result, many people are overweight, crave sugar and other carbohydrates, experience bouts of depression, get frequent headaches, and have vague muscle aches and pain. All of these maladies are correctable by raising brain serotonin levels; 5-HTP facilitates this process.

Folic Acid: Folic acid, also called folate or folacin, is a B vitamin with a solid reputation for protecting against birth defects and heart disease.

Folic acid also helps combat other ailments, such as depression, Alzheimer's disease, and certain types of cancer. Many people have a folic acid deficiency because it is easily lost through cooking or the processing of food.

Folic acid is often deficient in those who are depressed, and taking a supplement may help. Studies of depressed people with low blood levels of folic acid show that taking it in supplement form can improve the effectiveness of antidepressants. Folic acid also appears to reduce the high levels of homocysteine associated with some forms of depression.

GABA (Gamma-Aminobutyric Acid): GABA is the most abundant neurotransmitter in the brain. It helps induce relaxation and sleep, acting as a natural tranquilizer. GABA has also shown to be helpful in controlling seizures.

Garlic: For centuries, garlic has been recognized around the world as a spice, a food, and an herbal folk remedy. Garlic helps fight heart disease, high cholesterol, and high blood pressure. It is also a natural antibiotic and combats respiratory infections.

Horsetail (Equisetum arvense): The name horsetail arose because it was thought that the plant's stalk resembled a horse's tail. Today, the most notable uses for horsetail are as a mild diuretic and as an astringent for the genitourinary system, providing relief for kidney stones and bladder infections. Scientists have even identified the compounds in horsetail that promote fluid loss (equisetonin and flavone glycosides). As a rich source of silica, horsetail is also touted for its ability to strengthen nails, hair, and teeth; the body requires silica to keep these connective tissues healthy and strong. Never take horsetail to reduce the swelling associated with poor kidney or heart function; both are potentially serious conditions that require careful medical monitoring.

Hyaluronic Acid: Hyaluronic acid is a component of connective tissue whose function is to cushion and lubricate. Hyaluronan occurs throughout the body in abundant amounts. Interestingly, the availability of zinc and magnesium has an impact on hyaluronic acid levels in the body, and magnesium and zinc deficiencies are known to be associated with many of the same symptoms associated with hyaluronic acid abnormalities, such as mitral valve prolapse and poor wound healing. The jury is still out on whether hyaluronic acid is linked to breast cancer, so be sure to check with your doctor first.

Inositol: Inositol is a close relative to sugar and is part of the B-complex vitamins. One of the most versatile nutrients for promoting brain wellness, a positive and relaxed outlook, and restful sleep, inositol is also one of the most crucial nutrients for promoting female hormonal health through its role in supporting optimal liver function. Inositol also helps maintain healthy serotonin metabolism, and by so doing helps treat many conditions that involve poor serotonin function. Take the powdered form for optimal dosing.

L-Carnitine: Carnitine is a nutrient that facilitates the body's ability to burn fats for energy. Optimizing carnitine levels has been found to have dramatic benefits for combating low energy, obesity, and fatigue. Controlled trials have demonstrated that carnitine increases weight loss by promoting optimal fat burning by the mitochondria. Carnitine also helps promote heart health, maintenance of healthy cholesterol levels, and sports endurance and recovery.

L-Glutamine: L-glutamine is a conditionally essential amino acid, which means that our body can produce it but under times of stress our needs increase. L-glutamine is the most widely used ulcer preventative in China and Japan. L-glutamine heals inflammation inside the intestinal wall, and ultimately boosts immune function. It helps stop diarrhea in patients who suffer from Crohn's disease or colitis, as well as those fighting the side effects of chemotherapy. L-glutamine also helps to maintain muscle mass. Use the powdered form for optimal dosing.

Licorice Root: Licorice *(Glycyrrhiza glabra)* is a flavorful herb that has been used in food and medicinal remedies for thousands of years. It helps the body adapt better to stress by supporting adrenal function. Licorice acts as a demulcent (a soothing, coating agent) to relieve respiratory ailments (such as allergies, bronchitis, colds, sore throats, and tuberculosis), stomach problems (including heartburn and gastritis), inflammatory disorders, skin diseases, and liver problems.

Lipoic Acid: Lipoic acid is an antioxidant that has been extensively researched for its applications in diabetes, blood sugar metabolism, heavy-metal detoxification, liver health, hepatitis, and diabetic neuropathy. Lipoic acid helps the body produce energy, thus fighting the aging process. It also optimizes the function of the insulin receptors, making it an essential nutrient for diabetics.

L-Lysine: L-lysine is an essential amino acid that cannot be manufactured by the human body; we can get L-lysine only through diet or supplementation. The human body benefits from L-lysine because it promotes absorption of calcium, which ultimately boosts immune function. Lysine is a wonderful natural remedy for people with cold sores, shingles, or genital herpes.

L-Theanine: L-theanine, an amino acid naturally found in tea, promotes relaxation. L-theanine helps increase GABA production in the body, creating an alert yet totally relaxed state of mind without drowsiness. It is estimated that a heavy tea drinker (six to eight cups a day) will consume between 200 and 400 mg of L-theanine daily.

Magnesium: Magnesium is the fourth most abundant mineral in the body and is essential to good health. Approximately 50 percent of total body magnesium is found in bone; the other half is found predominantly inside the cells of tissues and organs. Magnesium helps maintain normal muscle and nerve function, keeps the heart rhythm steady, supports a healthy immune system, and keeps bones strong. Because of this, magnesium serves well as a muscle relaxant and aids in relieving muscular and menstrual cramps. Magnesium also helps regulate blood sugar levels, promotes normal blood pressure, and is known to be involved in energy metabolism and protein synthesis.

Maitake D: Maitake D-fraction, an extract from the maitake mushroom, is a bioactive compound composed of uniquely branched polymers that provide immune-system and cell support. Several studies suggest that maitake D-fraction works by activating immune-system messenger cells such as macrophages and cytokines. Beta-glucan, a type of polysaccharide (string of sugar molecules) obtained from several types of mushrooms, is being studied as a treatment for cancer and as an immune-system stimulant.

Micellized Vitamin A: Micellized vitamin A is the most easily absorbed form of vitamin A. It is extremely safe, even in high doses, because it bypasses the liver. Micellized vitamin A is extremely useful when you need to take a therapeutic dose of vitamin A to treat asthma, lung infections, acne, skin conditions, or immune disorders. The micellization process involves turning vitamin A into water-soluble micelles, which are ultimately much more easily absorbed across the gut wall.

MSM (Methylsulfonylmethane): MSM is an organic sulfur-containing nutrient that occurs naturally in the environment and in the human body. Sulfur is necessary for the structure of every cell in the body. Hormones, enzymes, antibodies, and antioxidants all depend on it. And because the body utilizes and expends it on a daily basis, sulfur must be continually replenished for optimal nutrition and health.

N-Acetyl Cysteine (NAC): NAC is an amino acid and a precursor to glutathione, the body's most powerful antioxidant. Studies have shown that NAC can help protect against such respiratory ailments as bronchitis, bronchial asthma, emphysema, and chronic sinusitis and may even help defend against lung damage caused by the cancer-causing chemicals in cigarette smoke. NAC has also been used effectively in treating inner-ear infections. Bodybuilders report that it helps them recover faster from their workouts.

Olive Leaf Extract: Derived from the leaves of the olive tree, olive leaf extract is an antibacterial, antiviral, and antiparasitic substance that will help fight off the common cold, as well as active herpes outbreaks. People taking blood thinners or antibiotics should exercise caution, as olive leaf extract could reduce the efficacy of both medications. For best results, look for capsules that contain 500 mg standardized to 20 percent oleuropein.

Omega-3s: Omega-3s are essential fatty acids found in fish and fish oil. About 15 percent of the alpha linoleic acid in flaxseed oil will also convert to omega-3s in the body of a healthy person. According to the National Research Council, more than sixty health conditions have been shown to benefit from essential fatty acid supplementation. Omega-3s help reduce systemic and localized inflammation; they also treat dry skin, depression, PMS and menstrual cramps, high cholesterol and triglycerides, and poor circulation. Wild Alaskan salmon, sardines, and krill are all excellent sources of omega-3s, as they are all naturally low in mercury.

Pancreatic Enzymes: In order to assimilate vitamins and nutrients from our food and supplements, we must be able to digest them properly. Pancreatic enzymes are critical for the digestion of proteins, fats, and carbohydrates. If you feel gassy and bloated after meals, are regularly constipated, or feel full after eating only a small quantity of food, you're a good candidate for digestive enzymes. Studies show that the foods in the typical American diet are devoid of natural enzymes and do little to help us secrete our own production of enzymes. Taking digestive enzymes will help you digest and absorb nutrients from your food, which is a large component of overall health.

Phosphatidylcholine: Phosphatidylcholine is the active ingredient in lecithin. Lecithin is a fatty substance needed for a wide variety of crucial bodily functions, such as building cell membranes and helping nutrients move in and out of cells. Phosphatidylcholine breaks down fat deposits in the body, making it valuable in the prevention of atherosclerosis and heart disease. It is also essential to the liver, and helps the liver remove toxins from the body.

Phosphatidylserine: Phosphatidylserine is vital to brain cell structure and function. It plays an important role in our neurotransmitter systems and in maintaining nerve connections in the brain. Phosphatidylserine not only helps boost cognitive performance and learning ability but also helps lower cortisol levels in the body brought on by stress or overexercising.

Probiotics: Natural, "good" bacteria that live in our intestines, helping the digestive tract and immune system stay healthy. Probiotics are found in most yogurts and are available in powdered or capsule form. Probiotics are most commonly sold under the names "acidophilus," "bifidus," or "lactobacillus." It is imperative to take them during and after a course of antibiotics so that you can replace what's been lost.

Quercetin: Quercetin is a bioflavonoid, one of a group of potent nutrients that are found in plants, fruits, vegetables, teas, apples, onions, and beans. Quercetin acts to inhibit the release of histamines during allergic reactions like eczema, asthma, and hay fever.

Spanish Black Radish: An herb that belongs to the phytonutrient-rich cruciferous family of vegetables, Spanish black radish has a natural antibiotic action and promotes systemic cleansing by activating the liver's primary detoxification mechanism.

St. John's Wort: The herb St. John's wort is beneficial in treating mild to moderate depression, seasonal affective disorder, mild anxiety, insomnia, stress, and viral infections such as herpes, chicken pox, and shingles. Check with your doctor before taking St. John's wort if you are on any type of prescription medication, and avoid excessive sunlight. Liquid tinctures of St. John's wort will be absorbed most effectively.

Taurine: Taurine is a conditionally essential amino acid, which means the body can make it but will require more under times of stress. Vegetarians who do not eat meat will need to supplement with taurine. It serves to protect the heart and lower blood pressure, and it also helps bile acids in the gallbladder clear cholesterol from the body. Taurine works in conjunction with vitamin B_6 as a safe diuretic that will not cause any loss or imbalance of minerals in the body.

Tea Tree Oil: Derived from the Australian tea tree, tea tree oil is a natural antiseptic, germicide, antibacterial, and fungicide. Many people use tea tree oil for acne, athlete's foot, cold sores, gum problems, and mosquito bites. The oils from the tea tree blend well with the skin's natural oils, so it is gentle yet effective.

Tyrosine: Tyrosine is a nonessential amino acid synthesized in the body from phenylalanine. It helps the body produce the brain neuro-transmitters epinephrine, norepinephrine, and dopamine. Tyrosine is also used to produce one of the major hormones, thyroxine, which plays an important role in controlling the metabolic rate, skin health, mental health, and growth. Tyrosine is specifically used to treat depression because it is a precursor for those neurotransmitters that are responsible for transmitting nerve impulses and are essential for preventing depression. Tyrosine may also be used as a mild appetite suppressant. Be sure to notify your doctor if you are taking tyrosine while on antidepressants, because tyrosine naturally raises dopamine levels in the brain and may decrease your need for medication.

Vitamin B_6: A water-soluble vitamin that is essential for good health, vitamin B_6 is needed for protein metabolism and red blood cell metabolism. The nervous and immune systems need vitamin B_6 to function efficiently. Vitamin B_6 is known to help naturally regulate water balance in the cells. It works in conjunction with taurine as a safe diuretic that does not cause any loss or imbalance of minerals in the body.

Vitamin D: Vitamin D is a fat-soluble steroid hormone that has long been known for its important role in regulating body levels of calcium and phosphorus and in the mineralization of bone. Vitamin D is even more important than calcium in building bone density, because it controls intestinal absorption of calcium. In addition to taking vitamin D orally, it is helpful to get fifteen minutes of sunshine at least three times per week to help your body make adequate amounts of vitamin D.

Wheat-Germ Oil: A rich source of vitamin E that is derived from the wheat berry. Vitamin E is a potent antioxidant that can help us make our sex hormones. It can be taken orally or inserted into the vagina at bedtime to relieve dryness.

Zinc: Zinc is an essential mineral that is found in almost every cell. It stimulates the activity of approximately one hundred enzymes, which are substances that promote biochemical reactions in your body. Zinc supports a healthy immune system, is essential for wound healing, helps maintain your sense of taste and smell, and is needed for DNA synthesis. Zinc is also a precursor for estrogen, progesterone, and testosterone.

RESOURCES

Culinary Support

Barefoot Contessa — www.barefootcontessa.com

Annemarie Colbin — www.foodandhealing.com

Nigella Lawson — www.nigella.com

Health and Fitness

American Social
Health Association — www.ashastd.org

Dr. Loren Cordain — www.thepaleodiet.com

Environmental Working
Group — www.ewg.org and
www.foodnews.org

Gregory Joujon-Roche — www.holisticfitness.com

Dr. Phil Maffetone — www.pccoach.com

Dr. Joseph Mercola — www.mercola.com

Geneen Roth — www.geneenroth.com

Neti Pots — www.thenetipot.com

The Nutrition Reporter — www.thenutritionreporter.com

Organic regulations — www.organicconsumers.org

Thyroid support — www.thyroid.about.com

Weston A. Price Foundation — www.westonaprice.org

Lifestyle and Beauty

Daily Candy   www.dailycandy.com

Devachan Salon   www.devachansalon.com

Juli B.   www.julib.com

Whole Foods

Gluten-free diet support   www.scdiet.com and
                              www.scdiet.org

Grass-fed beef   www.grassfedorganics.com

Raw, organic milk   www.realmilk.com

Soy   www.soyonlineservice.co.nz

Wild Alaskan salmon   www.vitalchoice.com

Fun Reading

Periel Aschenbrand   *The Only Bush I Trust Is My Own*

Dianne Brill   *Boobs, Boys, and High Heels*

Judy Ford   *Single: The Art of Being Satisfied,
                              Fulfilled, and Independent*

Anka Radakovich   *The Wild Girls Club* and
                              Sexplorations

Karen Salmansohn   *Even God is Single*

SARK   *Succulent Wild Woman*

ACKNOWLEDGMENTS

To help a girl get Gorgeous, it truly takes a village:

Celeste Fine, for believing in my product and launching it to the universe. Celeste, you are Gorgeous inside and out, and your moral support, can-do attitude, and furtherance of my naughty ways were a joy to work with. Thank you is not enough for all you've done—I'm forever grateful!

Jodi Warshaw, for bringing my text to places I'd never dreamed of. Your mind is divine, and I thank you from the bottom of my heart for your endless patience, creativity, and ability to work with a New York Virgo!

A heartfelt thank-you goes to Kate Prouty, for her editorial suggestions.

Jeff Harris, for graciously contributing his time and photographic talents for the cover photos. I am proud to call you my friend!

Special thanks to Lisa Dubrow, brainiac extraordinaire. You are part brass, part class, and all woman. Roar!

Kella England, for believing in something she'd never even seen, and then pitching my book to David Vigliano anyway. You were instrumental in making this all happen.

Robert Crayhon, my mentor and friend, who helped me conceptualize the initial outline for the book.

Gary Lasneski, who has enriched my practice and my life with his otherworldly knowledge, enabling me to bring great healing to my clients.

Lorraine Massey, for helping me to project my project and never taking no for an answer.

My amazing parents, Florence and Larry, and mother-in-law, Marcia, and the rest of my family: Steve, Andrea, Leo, Robert, Shari, David, Jodi, Dara, and Debby, for their endless support, encouragement, and love.

My incredibly sexy, sassy, Gorgeous friends—Nicole, Poopsie, Sandi, Melanie, Kathryn, Rachel, Diana, Karen, Barbara, Julie, two Judys, as well as so many others—for cheering me on, understanding my absences, and always helping me out "in the name of research." I am incredibly lucky to have you in my life.

Last but not least, my fabulous husband and rock, Jeremy, who selflessly stood by my side from start to finish, rooted for me the entire way, and fed me words when they wouldn't come. I think I'm the luckiest girl in the world to have you in my life. You are an extraordinary treasure.

INDEX